If You Love It,
it will GROW

a guide to healthy, beautiful natural hair

PHOENYX AUSTIN, M.D.

If You Love It, It Will Grow: A Guide To Healthy, Beautiful Natural Hair by Phoenyx Austin, M.D.

Website: drphoenyx.com

Email: dr.phoenyx@gmail.com

ISBN 978-0-9848630-0-6   ISBN 978-0-9848630-1-3

Printed in the United States of America

Published by Phoenyx Austin

This book contains information obtained from published literature and research from highly regarded resources. Reasonable efforts have been made to publish currently available, reliable information. The author and publisher, however, assume no responsibility for the validity of data contained herein or consequences for its use or misuse.

Although every effort has been made to properly reference, acknowledge and attribute respective owners of copyrighted material, the publisher and author is glad to acknowledge any omissions or clarifications brought to our attention in future editions and reprints of this book.

MEDICAL DISCLAIMER

The reader should use their best judgment when utilizing information in this book. Dr. Phoenyx Austin, the author, is not a professional hair care provider. The author's advice and information is based upon years of experience in caring for her own hair. Furthermore, the medical and nutritional information in this book is provided as an informational resource only, and is not to be used or relied on for any diagnostic or treatment purposes. The information in this book should not be used as a substitute for professional consultation, diagnosis and/or treatment. Please consult your health care provider before making any nutritional or healthcare decisions. The information in this book is intended for education, entertainment and does not create a patient-physician relationship. The author shall have neither responsibility nor liability to any person or entity with respect to any loss or damage alleged to be caused directly or indirectly by the advice or information contained in this book.

To God who gave me the gift. And to every beautiful brown skin girl who gave me the inspiration.

ACKNOWLEDGMENTS

I'D LIKE TO THANK...

My Mommy and Daddy for their love and the sacrifices they've made to give me every opportunity for success.

My extended family and dear friends for contributing an invaluable amount of constructive criticism, emotional support and inspiration for this book.

My editor, who worked magic in the background, took my book from draft to final, and most importantly, who thankfully doesn't believe in the 5 business day workweek.

I'd also like to acknowledge the school and individuals that were instrumental in me achieving one of my greatest goals in life:

To my outstanding alma mater, Meharry Medical College

To the late and great Dr. Pamela C. Williams, Executive Vice Dean of Meharry Medical College

To the dynamic duo- Dr. Dexter Stallworth and Dr. Reed Murtagh

ABOUT THE AUTHOR

Dr. Phoenyx Austin is a certified Sports Medicine Specialist, best-selling author, and the creator of Dr. Phoenyx brand nutritional supplements for healthy hair and fit body. Order Dr. Phoenyx's advanced nutritional supplements, *Beauty&Body Protein* for Healthy Hair and Fit Body, and *Natural Beauty* for Healthy Hair, Skin & Nails at DRPHOENYX.COM.

CONTENTS

FOREWORD

For black women, the topic of hair is often deeply personal, political and far too often painful. Outside of our community, there is great confusion about it (think: the cringe worthy *"Can I touch it?"* and *"How do you get it like that?"* inquiries from even well-intentioned non-black friends). Sometimes our men even reveal issues, hang-ups and ignorance regarding our hair (think: the well-intentioned documentary *"Good Hair"*).

Despite decades of *"Black is Beautiful"* campaigns and sloganism, many sisters see their hair as a challenge, not source of pride. However, the natural hair movement of recent years has created a surge in hair-related pride. Black women have created sister circles, websites and social networks devoted solely to the celebration and care of our tresses in its natural state. Buzz over black women and natural hair is everywhere, but the conversation is not always an easy one.

You see, as we have raised a glass to the sister who wears her 'fro big and proud, many sisters who dare to continue loving their straight and/or permed tresses have been shunned; some have even had their "Blackness" challenged. Is the hot comb not yet authentically Black? Is the perm box not as much a part of our culture as the Afro pick? We have to recognize that even as we celebrate the acceptance and love of our God-given hair textures that "real" Black aesthetics are as diverse and different as the shades of our skin.

I consider myself quite lucky to have been raised by parents who made it quite clear that my natural hair was "enough." I was denied the perm I requested in middle school and even press-outs were reserved for special occasions only. My greatest hang-ups about my hair came from my own inability to properly care for it as a rebellious teen with a penchant for bright colors and the insistence of my classmates that my hair was nice, but that it would probably look "real pretty" if I would just straighten it. As an adult, I've worn dreads, braids, wigs and many variations of the big bushy 'fro. I love my natural hair texture and I love the look of a fresh wrap and set. Why? Because my hair is healthy and well cared for. I'm good to my hair and it is good to me.

However, I recognize that for far too many sisters, a positive relationship with one's hair is not a given, but a destination. If you are still looking to build that sort of love for your own tresses, you've come to the right place.

Much of my enthusiasm about this book comes from Dr. Phoenyx's refusal to throw our sisters who chemically straighten their hair under the bus. She offers healthy solutions for natural hair care that can be adopted even by those who are quite content using chemicals to straighten their hair. Dr. Phoenyx has also resisted this new trend of making "curly" or "multi-racial"-looking hair the center of the natural hair conversation and has instead used the term "afro-textured" to refer to the multi-textural goodness that comes from the scalps of black women across the globe.

Here, you will find a holistic approach to hair care and a very straight-forward premise: *if you love your hair, it will grow.* If you treat your hair with care, it will be healthy and strong. If longer hair is your goal, you can achieve that with proper nurturing. We must stop treating Black hair as a problem to solve and instead, have a positive image of our hair. It isn't enough to only love your hair when it's "done" or when you have a fresh press. To have the hair you want, you should love the hair you were given and find healthy ways to make it work. ***If You Love It, It Will Grow*** isn't simply a clever title…it's the truth!

There are many folks who want to give black women advice for the sake of a paycheck or self-promotion (or both!). Dr. Phoenyx, however, is a proven expert in afro-textured hair care and is presenting this information in a loving, altruistic way. Her work speaks for itself: as a physician with a strong educational base in both traditional and alternative medicine, she has a firm understanding of how our hair lives and grows. As a writer and media personality, she has shared this wisdom with audiences across the country. If that isn't enough, she also has a head of glorious, healthy natural hair (and a testimony behind it) to prove that she isn't simply talking the talk … she's walking the walk!

Self-love and care is the key to healthy, beautiful hair and this book can help you understand that in ways that few others have. I hope that you enjoy *If You Love It, It Will Grow* as much as I have and that Dr. Phoenyx's expert advice is as good to your afro-textured hair as it has been to mine!

Jamilah Lemieux
Content Editor, *EBONY.com*

INTRODUCTION

If you are a woman who has been searching for a comprehensive resource that explains how to grow and maintain healthy, longer afro-textured hair in a simple and straightforward way, then this book is for you! But before we get to all of that, let me tell you a bit more about who I am and what I hope to share with you.

My name is Dr. Phoenyx Austin, and some of you may already be familiar with my articles and videos on fitness, natural beauty and healthy living topics. Overall, I love sharing advice and tips with women on how we can achieve both our beauty *and* body goals by practicing healthy habits like exercising regularly and maintaining a healthy diet. And every now and again, I get questions like, *"What should I do to grow my hair long?"* or *"What vitamins should I take to grow my hair?"* or *"How do you take care of your hair Dr. Phoenyx?"*

After getting so many inquiries about hair, and realizing I had so much information to share on the topic, it just made perfect sense to write a book about hair care. Yes, I am an MD who knows a lot about health and hair, but I also want to emphasize that first and foremost I'm just a woman who wants to feel good and look good. And having the hair I want is a significant part of that. So while writing this book, I frequently referred back to all the knowledge I've acquired through the years of professional training, and being that I have degrees in both psychology and medicine, this book will be part introspective, part medical and even a bit scientific at times.

That said, this book will also be very personal. And believe me when I say that I thought long and hard about what I wanted to include in this book, and when I first conceptualized it, I knew that I wanted to get personal about my own hair journey because there is a deeper message that I want to share..

I should start by saying that I am a woman who has learned to love her hair. For many years, I struggled with my hair. I wanted it to be beautiful, I wanted it to be healthier, and I wanted it to be longer. But I could never manage to achieve all three of these things. I was utterly confused as to why because in my mind I was doing everything I *thought* I needed to do for my hair to grow. As time went on, I eventually grew to dislike my hair and even viewed it as inferior to other hair types. For years I struggled with hair that left me very frustrated and very unhappy.

This was the way I felt about my hair for many years until a few life experiences and lots of education led to a change in perspective. It was when I made a conscious decision to change the way I viewed my hair, and started taking care of my hair, that I started to see the results I wanted. Simply put, I learned to love my hair. Learning to love my hair is what led to developing a personal hair philosophy and embracing hair practices that have helped me reach my hair goals. Now, my hair is healthy and the length that I have always desired.

So much of who we are and how we perceive ourselves is intricately tied to our hair. This book is about growing hair to longer lengths, but is also about a deeper message; a message of self-love and self-acceptance. For many women, hair is not just hair. There is a great interconnectedness between how women feel about their hair and how they feel about themselves. In many ways, our hair is an extension of who we are.

Thank you so much for taking the time to read my book. I hope you find the information in it to be extremely helpful as you work towards your hair goals. It's always a great feeling when someone, man or woman, randomly stops you in the store or on the street and tells you that they love your hair. But it is an even better feeling when YOU look in the mirror and can say the same to yourself.

When growing hair to longer lengths, you just need to start from a place of love. Love is patient. Love is kind. Love is nurturing. Love is cherishing. Love is protecting. If you love it, it will grow!

WHAT TO EXPECT FROM THIS BOOK

This book is about growing longer and healthier afro-textured hair. So, if those are your hair goals, then you've picked up the right book.

In the beginning I'll share my hair story, and I'll be blunt, I've had a pretty rocky relationship with my hair. Still, I want to share my hair struggles and triumphs with you. Many of us have a story to tell when it comes to our hair- maybe you'll even identify with a few of my hair experiences. Ultimately, the purpose of sharing my hair story is to show you where I came from and where I am now.

After my hair story, I will get into the nitty-gritty of hair and hair growth. We'll cover topics like how hair grows, what hair needs in order to be healthy, how hair becomes damaged, and how you can prevent hair damage. We will also cover how you can best use nutrition for hair growth, how to select commercial products, how to set up a healthy hair regimen, how to treat scalp issues, and many, many other topics that will help you achieve maximum health and maximum length with your hair. The information in this book comes from my perspective as a doctor and as a woman with afro-textured hair.

I wanted to make this book about growing healthy and long hair. Everything you need to know about that is included in this book. My book is not about styling hair, which is why I did not include a bunch of pictures of different hairstyles. The internet is a great place to find pictures and videos on how to style hair- if that's what you desire. This book is about growth, so if you've been looking for information on how to grow longer, healthy afro-textured hair- keep reading! This book is definitely for you.

CHAPTER 1

MY HAIR STORY

*"Eventually I knew what my hair wanted; it wanted to be itself... to be
left alone by anyone, including me, who did not love it as it was."*
– ALICE WALKER

I got my first relaxer in kindergarten. I didn't know *why* it was being done-
and when I asked the question, I was simply told that I *"needed it"* in order
to make my hair more manageable.

Every eight weeks, and always on a Saturday morning, my mom and I
would take a trip to the beauty salon. I started going to the beauty salon
when I was very young, not too long after my parents and I arrived in
the United States from Panama. I'm Afro-Latina and come from a long
lineage of men and women raised on West Indian values. My mother, a
very conservative woman, sought to instill many of those values in me;
one of those values being that a little girl should never leave the house
without looking *"presentable."* Every day my mother would inspect my
clothes and style my hair. When I was five, she began booking me regular
appointments for a relaxer, deep conditioning, blow-dry, trim and style.

While I understood why my mother wanted me to look nice, I really hated
the process, particularly when it came to my hair. I hated the relaxer, as
well as the occasional scalp burns that came with it. I loathed the salon's
smell of chemicals and burnt hair. I disliked the loud buzz from the
hooded blow dryers and the uncomfortable heat from the curling irons.

Most of all, I hated that doing my hair took so much damn time. I can still remember my desperate pleas, *"Mommy! Can't I just stay home and watch The Smurfs, please? I want to watch cartoons! And why does it take so long to get my stupid hair done anyway?!?"*

Up until the age of five, Saturday mornings were for fun and cartoons. Now, they were spent in a salon. I began to hate how my hair infringed upon other aspects of my life. I was a huge tomboy and quite frankly, hair was not a priority of mine. You could usually find me climbing trees, swimming, riding my bike through muddy ditches, or skinning my knees. Those were my priorities. I remember coming home one day from an evening of usual horseplay. My hair looked a hot mess and my mom and dad couldn't resist laughing. They told me I looked like I had just stuck my finger in an electrical socket. But I just shrugged and laughed. As wild as my hair appeared to others, I never thought much of it. I was more concerned with being a kid and having fun. It was my belief that only silly girls and silly women worried more about their hair than enjoying life.

Then something began to change. Though I initially hated the experience, as time went on, I actually grew to embrace the salon visits. I began to really enjoy the compliments I received when my hair was freshly straightened and styled. OK, and of course there was a certain boy in my third grade class that kept me primping in the mirror a little more than usual.

Overall, I liked being thought of as pretty. All women with long, straight hair were considered attractive, and I wanted to be pretty just like them. On top of that, I wasn't oblivious to the negative comments and jokes that were openly made about natural hair. I regularly heard the *"your hair is so nappy,"* *"buckshots,"* and *"beadie bead"* jokes. I most certainly did not want to be on the receiving end of those quips. I did not want to be teased by other children or scrutinized by adults. I wanted to be thought of as beautiful. I wanted to be like the women around me, like the women on TV, and the women pictured on the relaxer box. I did not want to be the butt of a joke. I did not want to be ugly, and I did not want to have *"nappy hair."* Consciously and subconsciously, I came to believe that getting my hair straightened was a necessity.

I eventually reasoned that salon visits, relaxers, curling irons, and blow dryers were all essential means to looking beautiful. It was just like my mother had said when she took me for my first relaxer: I *"needed it."* I didn't like the process of becoming beautiful, but if I wanted to be beautiful, I would just have to suck it up. This was the path to beauty, so I did what I needed to do.

The years went by and eventually I entered into high school. I had become a budding young woman, and was now totally responsible for my own hair. My hair came down to the middle of my back and I enjoyed having long hair, but maintenance was another issue. I was now in my teenage years and fully aware of the constant conundrum of wanting to look good while also being in a regular state of hair vigilance. Sweat, water and wind were my biggest hair adversaries. I did everything possible to avoid them, even to the detriment of my health, happiness, and sanity.

Though I loved going to the beach, I avoided the water. Though I loved sports, I became less active because I worried about sweating my perm out. I loved being outdoors, but I would avoid going outside if it was humid, rainy, or windy. I would also go bananas if someone rolled down the car windows while we were driving. It was truly hilarious at times, but still very dysfunctional. I didn't realize it then, but I had literally become a prisoner to my own hair.

During my high school years, I recall one of my girlfriends deciding to cut off her relaxed hair. Throughout high school she wore her hair in a small Afro. She was the only person I knew who wore her in its natural state. Our parents were friends and I would constantly hear her mom talk about how her daughter *"needed"* to get a relaxer. Some classmates would also tease her about her *"nappy hair."* But, regardless of what others said, she continued to proudly wear her hair in its natural state. She and I would hang out sometimes and I would envy her confident and carefree attitude. I never probed too much about her hair, but I would often wonder what it would be like to be free of my relaxer as well. I wanted the freedom she seemed to have and I admired the beauty in her uniqueness. But all that admiration still wasn't enough to ignore my body-image issues or the social stigma of natural hair. I was very fearful. And though my chemically processed hair was a growing source of discontent, I still felt prettier, and even safer, with a relaxer.

Eventually, I entered college and became a pre-med student with barely enough time to eat, sleep, or even do my hair. I kept getting relaxers and also graduated to more heat styling and tons of product use. By the end of freshman year, the health of my hair had rapidly declined. I had tons of breakage and I was tired of dealing with my hair.

One day in physics class, I took notice of a beautiful brown-skin girl with long, flowing hair that draped down the back of her seat. She was sitting directly in front of me and would occasionally shake her head from side to side, sending waves of chocolate hair flowing back and forth. I stared at her hair, at one point even wanting to reach out and touch it, although I knew better. I knew I couldn't touch, but I could most certainly stare- and that's exactly what I did. For most of the fifty-minute lecture, I found myself completely fixated on her hair.

Once class was dismissed, I gently tapped her shoulder. She whipped her head around, and a few strands of her hair lightly brushed against my outstretched hand.

"Wow, your hair is gorgeous. How did you grow it so long?" I asked.

She smiled and replied, *"Thank you, but this is a weave."*

I was totally shocked. It looked so real. I then told her about my hair troubles and how I wanted to grow longer hair. She said that I just needed to give my hair a *"rest."* She raved about how fabulous weaves were for styling versatility. She also said they were a great way to protect hair from the damaging effects of daily maintenance. According to her, a weave would be the perfect way to grow my hair to longer lengths.

Honestly, it didn't take much convincing. Her hair looked great and I was desperate. She gave me the number to her stylist (a fellow undergrad student who did hair out her dorm room for extra cash). I was so ecstatic and thanked her profusely. Before I even made it out of the lecture hall, I was on my cell phone making the earliest appointment possible to get my hair done.

Needless to say, my first weave experience started out great. Within a couple of days, I had a full head of long, flowing hair just like the brown skin girl in my class. I was whipping it back and forth. You couldn't tell me I didn't look fly! I had long, full hair again, and I was getting compliments. It was all so fabulous! As far as I was concerned, weaves were one of the best inventions of all time- right below fried chicken and waffles.

Sometimes when I think back to the whole weave experience, I can't help but laugh at how naïve I was. I literally put a whole extra layer of hair on my head and allowed myself to totally forget about my actual hair growing underneath. Deep down I didn't want to concern myself with the hair growing from my scalp, so I simply covered it up. I even became quite sporadic with cleansing and conditioning my actual hair. All I saw was my weave and nothing else. And as funny as these memories are, the experience also speaks to how I wanted to disconnect from my hair.

I happily carried on with my *new* hair but within a month my nappy new growth had become very obvious against my silky straight weave. To remedy this issue, I quickly made an appointment to have my hair redone. It was probably one of the worst times I could've picked to do it. We were in the middle of midterms. Every student was stressed and sleep deprived. But I couldn't go another week without getting my hair done.

It was a Wednesday, 2 days before my midterm, and I was up late helping my student stylist hunt around her messy dorm room for a pair of scissors. There were textbooks, loose-leaf paper, and clothes everywhere. She eventually found a random pair of scissors and got to work at removing my tracks.

Snip- snip- snip.

She worked quickly with the scissors. A few tracks fell. I scratched my stiff and dry roots. She then took a fine-toothed comb and unbraided my cornrows. I watched her through a handheld mirror and winced at how dull and dirty my hair looked. I must've looked visibly disgusted.

"That's normal. Just go wash your hair and come back early in the morning. I'll redo your hair." She was very nonchalant.

When she was done unbraiding, I immediately threw a scarf over my head and went home. I hit the shower and stood under the cascade of warm water. I then poured a massive amount of shampoo in my hands and started scrubbing my hair. The first rinse sent a stream of brownish water spiraling down the drain. I lathered and rinsed my hair once more. I looked down at the shower floor and it was covered with strands of hair. I immediately felt a bit nervous, but calmed myself. They were *obviously* strands from the weave.

After conditioning my hair, I exited the shower and got to work on blow drying. As I pulled the comb through my wet hair and moved the blow dryer around my head, I took immediate notice at how jagged and thin the ends of my hair looked. My hair was only semi-dry when it became quite apparent that the hair on the bathroom floor was actually my own. *Did she also cut my hair while removing my weave?!?* I stared at my reflection in the mirror. My hair now looked like someone had taken a mini weed whacker to it. I was pissed!

The next day I was forced to get my hair cut. The stylist suggested a short, angled bob, *"It will look really good on you. You definitely have the face for it. Not everyone can wear this style."*

She could see how upset I was and was trying to console me. I didn't want such a drastic cut and she did try to offer other suggestions. In the end she basically told me that the damage from the chemicals, the heat, and now the weave, would require that I take several inches off of my ends. So, I let her cut my hair. When she was through, my hair ended up being shorter than it had ever been in my entire life. I couldn't even pull it back into a ponytail.

I must admit that as time went on, I actually came to like my haircut. It was flattering and easy to maintain. But deep down, I still desired longer hair.

Not too long after the whole weave fiasco I began to notice a few natural-haired women on campus. I had always been told that Black hair without a relaxer would be *"unmanageable"* and even *"ugly."* This made relaxers seem like the logical choice for someone who wanted healthy and long hair. But as time went on, that logic soon started to make less and less sense.

Contrary to what I had been conditioned to believe, I found that the natural-haired women at my university had some of the healthiest and fullest looking hair that I'd ever seen. Some women had big Afros and some had teeny-weeny Afros. Some had long twists and others had short locs. There were so many lovely types and textures of hair, with many different lengths. Every woman looked gorgeous and there was some-thing so cool about the way they wore their natural hair so confidently. I often wondered if my hair could ever look like theirs.

From time to time I'd ask a few of these women about their hair. They all seemed to say the same thing; they loved how much freer and happier they felt with natural hair. Conversation after conversation, I grew more and more certain that I wanted the peace that they had.

In time I actually stopped relaxing my hair, but I started regularly using heat to straighten my new growth. At one point I had been relaxer-free for about six months but I felt no more "liberated" than when I was chemically straightening my hair. My hair was still stressing me out, I was experiencing a lot of breakage, and there were many times that I strongly considered going back to relaxers.

It was now the summer of 2005 and I was on vacation in Jamaica with a few friends. We were on day two of our seven-day trip when I decided to risk missing a complimentary breakfast of ackee, saltfish and dumplings to spend an extra hour in the bathroom trying to fix my hair. I had forgotten to wrap it the previous night after a day of beaching and night of clubbing. My stomach grumbled and I was very agitated at the thought of missing breakfast. Still, as hungry as I was, there was no way I was leaving the hotel room with my hair looking like a rabid Chihuahua had gone to war with it.

I washed my hair and it was almost 11 am when I finally finished blow-drying, flat ironing, and curling my hair. I then finished things up with a ton of hair spray and oil sheen. After sufficiently burning an extra hole in the ozone layer with my hair products, I finally left the hotel room. I was in a mad rush down the stairs to the dining hall. As I ran, I could feel a heavy cloud of humid air descend upon me like a warm, wet blanket. I paused to look at my reflection through one of the hotel room windows. To my shock and dread, the humidity had completely ravaged my hair.

In less than 5 minutes my hair had been reduced to a partially limp, partially frizzy mess. It was a wrap. My hair looked like crap. And after all that work! I sighed and my stomach grumbled violently. Realizing that there wasn't much I could do, I simply muttered a few colorful, one-syllable words and pulled my hair back into a bun. I cursed my hair *and* Jamaica.

On the fourth day of our trip, I sat on the sand and caught glimpse of a young woman with the most beautiful locs I had ever seen. At one point she ran into the ocean and began splashing around with her boyfriend. They horsed around for a few minutes and afterwards she ran back to the beach to rinse her hair under one of the public showers. I watched her and thought about how nice it would be to get in and out of the water just like her. It seemed like every day in Jamaica was a struggle to find a happy medium where I could have a good time, while not messing up my hair. On top of that, every trip to the beach translated to over an hour of work on my hair. Eventually I was exhausted with it all, so much so that I began to stay out of the water.

I climbed onto my beach chair, took a sip of my slushy tropical drink, closed my eyes and let the rays of the sun warm my skin. Eventually the cocktail kicked in and my thoughts trailed off. I was almost asleep when one of my friends sneaked up, scooped me up onto his shoulder and hauled me off towards the ocean. He was at a brisk jog and I saw the water approaching us. I immediately panicked at the thought of getting my hair wet. I was kicking and shouting loudly for him to put me down, but he ignored my pleas.

"You're getting in this water girl!" He laughed and held me tight.

I put up a good struggle to get loose, but he and his six-foot three frame were easily able to carry me despite my kicks and flailing arms. In no time he waist deep in the ocean and I knew what was to come. As feared, he tossed me into the water like a rag doll. I gulped in saltwater and gasped for air. I splashed and stumbled around, trying to catch my footing among the waves. I felt out of breathe from all the shouting but still had enough air in my lungs to begin cussing him out for messing up my hair. He just laughed and tried to hold me in the water. After many slaps on his head and punches to his chest, I was able to get loose from his grip. I did eventually laugh too, especially after I realized how crazy I must've looked.

33

A few minutes later I made my exit from the water. On the way back to my beach chair I once again caught a glimpse of the same young woman with the gorgeous locs. She was standing alone by the bar. I began to walk towards her and was just a few feet behind her when she suddenly turned around and we made eye contact.

"I love your hair!" I blurted out.

She smiled and thanked me for the compliment. I asked her many questions about her hair and found out that she used to have relaxed hair too. She asked if I was thinking about going natural myself. I told her that I had stopped relaxing my hair, but was considering going back. Deep down I wanted to completely stop, but for some reason I kept holding on. I had gotten so used to straightening my hair and it was my security blanket. I also knew nothing about natural hair care. I rambled on and on. It was like I was having a therapy session with a complete stranger. She listened intently and offered as much advice as she could. Like the other women, she also loved how liberating it was to be free from chemical straightening. She was happy and truly loved her hair. I, on the other hand, was growing more and more frustrated and ashamed of my hair by the second.

As I stood there ogling her hair she must've caught wind of my emotional funk because she gently placed her hand on my arm and smiled, *"If you want to go natural, just do it girl! You'll look gorgeous either way."*

At that moment my eyes began to well with tears. My face started to feel hot and my vision was getting blurry. I quickly forced a smile, thanked her and made my way back to my beach chair before she could notice. On the way back I brushed away my tears and took a seat to compose myself. I was in shock that I had become so emotional in front of a complete stranger. I didn't realize until that moment how truly unhappy I was with my hair. I just sat there on my beach chair, silent and stewing. Not too long after, my friends were out of the water and we were on our way back to the hotel.

As we made our way up the sandy paved road and shanty shops, everyone chatted about how much fun they were having and how excited they were to be in Jamaica. I, on the other hand, wasn't in the same chipper mood. I was in a daze, a deep emotional funk. My friend asked me what was wrong, and I made up an excuse of being hungry and tired.

When we finally reached the hotel room, I made a dash to the bathroom and started to get ready. It was ten after six and I needed to start my hair ritual. I grabbed my huge arsenal of hair products and after a quick shower, jumped in front of the mirror and got to work. I piled on hair product, combed, brushed, blow-dried, flat-ironed and did everything in my power to get my hair looking right. I still remember the smell of burnt hair and the countless broken strands on the bathroom sink and floor. At one point, I stopped and stared at myself in the mirror. My hair was a limp, dull, tattered and damaged mess. It was hopeless. All I could do was just stand there and stare.

A few seconds later my girlfriend called out from the next room to see if I was almost ready.

I didn't answer her.

I just stood in front of the mirror, staring at the chemical and heat-damaged mess on my head. I didn't know where to begin or when it would all end. I hated my hair. I hated the reflection of the woman staring back at me. I thought back to that young woman on the beach and how much I envied her. I felt a wave of helplessness, confusion and sadness wash over me. I stared at myself wondering, *why am I doing this to myself?*

My girlfriend tapped on the bathroom door and I knew I couldn't stay in there pondering that question forever. I once again tied my hair in a bun and went to dinner with my friends.

After dinner I went back to my hotel and sat silently on the bed. I pulled out my journal and started to write. I also went back into the bathroom, looked at myself in the mirror and forced myself to answer that very question that had haunted me in the bathroom before dinner.

Why am I doing this to myself?

I wrote and I cried. I was tired of it all. I wanted to stop torturing myself. I wanted to stop being fearful. I wanted to stop hating my hair. But most importantly, I wanted to be happy in my skin.

For many years I did not love my hair and for many years I desired hair that wasn't my own. I was taught that chemicals and heat were the way to achieve what I thought I desired, but all of it came at the high price of my freedom and the ability to be myself. I couldn't be the girl who loved to hit the beach. I couldn't be the girl who loved to get caught in the rain. I was no longer that little girl who thought fussing over hair was silly. I had become someone else, someone unrecognizable to myself. Everything now revolved around my hair. My hair had literally taken over my life, and I hated my hair for that.

To make things worse, I was still never able to grow my hair to the length I always wanted. My hair was always damaged, constantly breaking, and Jamaica had literally become *my* breaking point. I had been in a constant battle with my hair, but I was finally ready to wave the white flag. It was when I chose to embrace my hair, and all that came with it, that I finally felt at peace.

A few days later my friends and I returned to Florida. The following day I called my friend (the same one who had thrown me into the ocean) and asked him to accompany me to his local barber. I told him that I was going to cut my hair off and explained why. I had mentally prepared myself for a barrage of criticisms. To my surprise, he was completely supportive. He told me that it was great that I had decided to stop being so obsessed with my hair. He also said he thought I'd look *"hot with a 'fro."*

He picked me up and drove us to the barbershop. We walked in, took a seat, and within a few minutes I was in the barber's chair. I explained what I wanted done.

"I want to cut off all my hair."

The barber looked at me. He didn't say a word, but his face clearly showed what he was thinking. He then looked at my friend, I guess for some sort of verification of my sanity. My friend smiled. The barber then looked at me again. I smiled and assured him that I was not *"crazy"* or *"going through something."* It was then that he began to press me on *why* I wanted to cut off my hair. He said I had *"good hair"* and that I would *"regret it."* I cringed as he spoke those words. For the next couple of minutes, we debated each other over **my hair**. He tried his hardest to convince me not to cut it and also added that I just needed to get a relaxer touch-up and my ends trimmed. Finally I, in somewhat of a child-like fit, put my hands on my hips and huffed, *"Look, if you don't do it, I'll just shave my head myself."*

He cracked a smile, shrugged his shoulders and picked up a pair of scissors.

The scissors moved quickly, and next came the buzzing of his clippers in my ears. My heart pounded as I watched my hair fall. It all felt like slow motion. I breathed deeply and stared at my reflection in the large mirror. The barber moved around my head with swiftness and precision. Within in a few minutes, all that remained attached to my scalp were a few inches of black, poofy hair.

The barber dusted off my shoulders, sprayed my hair with a watery solution, shaped up my poof, spun my chair around, and handed me a small mirror so I could get a 360° view. I looked at my reflection, wide-eyed and speechless. I then looked up at my friend. He stepped closer and placed his hands in my hair. He gently scrunched my curls and kinks like a baker kneading dough. Then he gently massaged my scalp with his fingertips. His touch felt like heaven. I had a big Kool-Aid grin plastered on my face and let my head fall backwards.

The barber shook his head, laughed at my giddiness and began sweeping up my hair. I asked him to place it in a large clear zip lock bag I had brought with me. I wanted to keep that bag of hair as a reminder. I had a newfound freedom and a newfound love for my hair. I promised myself that I would never again hate any part of me. I would always remember that day and the growth that came from it.

That was almost seven years ago. And though I could say that the journey to *fully* loving my hair ended there, that would certainly not be true. In fact, my journey had just begun. Yes, I had found love for my hair and I was happy to be free, but I still needed to acquire knowledge and develop skills to take my hair to the healthy lengths I wanted. Simply cutting off my hair didn't magically give me all the tools I needed to grow longer and healthy hair. I needed greater action and commitment to accomplish that. So, I began learning more about hair care and speaking with more natural-haired women.

Natural hair did in fact come with its own unique challenges and requirements. I learned that simply having natural hair did not automatically lead to longer hair, especially if I kept using blow dryers, flat irons, and other things that would irreparably damage my hair. I learned that if I wanted longer and healthy hair, I would need to totally change the way I treated it, as well as the rest of my body. I say that because I came to learn that my hair is a reflection of my inner state of health. I learned how nutrition, exercise, and even stress can affect hair growth. I also learned about making better product choices for my hair and how to care for my hair on a daily basis. I basically learned to look at hair growth from a holistic standpoint.

Eventually I began treating my hair better than I had treated it in my entire life. It was then that I came to view my healthy hair growth as due to one major factor—*love*. When I loved my hair, I cherished it. When I cherished my hair, I protected it from harm. This is when my hair began to thrive and grow to the healthy, long lengths that I desired. My experiences and observations then gave birth to a new hair philosophy: *If you love it, it will grow.* When I loved it, my hair began to grow!

CHAPTER 2

WHAT DOES 'IF YOU LOVE IT, IT WILL GROW' REALLY MEAN?

I decided to title my book *If You Love It, It Will Grow* because I want to highlight what hair needs to be healthy, and what it needs to grow to longer lengths. Women are constantly inquiring about what they need to do for healthy, longer hair. The answer is quite simple. No matter how you slice it, your hair ultimately needs one key thing if you want to accomplish these goals—love!

So now you may be thinking, *"What does love mean?"*

Well for me, love takes on several meanings. Love is nurturing. Love is patient. Love is commitment. Love is protection from harm. In fact, I consider the whole process of growing hair to be a *"labor of love."* Make no mistake, the whole process takes a certain degree of work. You will have to be nurturing, committed, patient and protective. This is how I approach my hair and I am certain that once you approach your hair the same way, you will also be able to achieve the growth you desire as well.

Now let me ask you this question: *Do you have trouble growing your hair to the length you want?*

If the answer to the above question is yes, I now want to ask you this question: *Do you love your hair?*

Really think about that second question.

If you don't love your hair, then unfortunately this book is not going to be of much use to you. You need to start loving your hair in order to achieve growth. Not loving your hair is a very slippery slope that ultimately leads to unhealthy hair habits and unrealistic hair expectations.

Though this book was inspired by personal experiences, I want to emphasize that "love" is not about natural versus relaxed hair. Love is all about caring for your hair so that it is the healthiest it can be to achieve maximum length. That stated, when you love something, you treat it right and make the best choices for it. This is the frame of mind you need to be in if you want this book to work. When you truly love something, like your hair (or anything for that matter) you will treasure it and make healthy choices to maintain it. When you love your hair, you will not be inclined to do things that are contrary to its health and growth. You cannot chronically neglect and damage your hair, *and then* expect it to grow to its maximum potential. That is what I would call unhealthy hair habits and an unrealistic expectation.

See where I'm coming from?

Loving your hair makes all the difference for growth potential. Please understand this. Love is where you always need to begin *and* end if you want your hair to grow.

CHAPTER 3
BASICS OF HAIR GROWTH

As much as we like to think of our hair as a fashion statement, the truth is that Mother Nature wasn't too concerned with how "hot" we'd look when she gave us a full head of hair. In fact, the hair on our head is actually designed for protection. Actually, *all* the hair on our body serves some role of protection.

Hair is designed to protect our scalp from overexposure to the sun. Hair is also a thermoregulator and prevents tremendous amounts of body heat from escaping through our skin. Even our eyebrows and eyelashes serve to protect our eyes from beads of sweat and dust particles. These are just a few examples of how our hair protects other parts of our body. It's just a lucky coincidence that our hair can make us look super cute too!

HAIR FOLLICLES & HAIR TYPING

The scalp is where hair growth begins. You cannot achieve healthy hair growth without a health scalp. Many women don't think of hair growth in these terms, but that's the way it works. In order to grow healthy hair, you have to maintain the health of your scalp.

Every hair on your head comes out through a single hair follicle in your scalp. The hair follicle is a very small structure that sits just below the surface of the skin. In fact, your entire body, not just your scalp, is literally covered in hair follicles. The average person will have millions of hair follicles with approximately 100,000 of those hair follicles on their head. The only places you won't find hair follicles or hair are on the palms of your hands and the soles of your feet.

Approximately 91% of the structure of your hair is protein, and the hair follicle itself produces this protein called keratin. In addition to keratin, hair is also composed of color pigment (i.e. melanin), vitamins, traces of minerals like zinc, and water. It sounds pretty straightforward, but the structure and composition of hair can get pretty complex. But for the purposes of this book I'm going to keep things simple in regards to growing hair to longer lengths. Quite simply, I want to emphasize **now** that of all the things that make up hair, there are two components that will greatly determine whether your hair is able to grow to healthy and longer lengths. Those two components are protein and water. I will explain why later.

WHAT MAKES HAIR NATURALLY CURLY VS. NATURALLY STRAIGHT?

There are several ways to categorize hair. One obvious way is whether it's curly or straight. Women often wonder what makes their hair naturally straight or naturally curly. Is it their genes or is it something else? What determines whether your hair will be curly or straight?

It's actually the shape of your hair follicle as well as the angle at which hair grows out of the follicle that will determine whether your hair is curly or straight. Straight hair grows vertically out of the hair follicle. Curly, wavy and kinky hair will grow out of the hair follicle at an angle. This angle of growth happens because women with straight hair have straight, l-shaped hair follicles, while women with curly hair have curved, c-shaped hair follicles.

One of the most simplistic systems for categorizing hair types was designed by Andrew Walker, a multi-Emmy award winning celebrity stylist. Mr. Walker developed his own Hair Type Classification System

(HTCS) to identify the various types of hair based on curl pattern. This system has been widely referenced to help women learn how to best care for their hair based on type. In his system Mr. Walker identifies 4 basic types of hair, which can be further broken down into subcategories such as Type 2a or 4b:

Type 1 - Straight Hair (hair without curl or wave pattern)

Type 2 - Wavy (hair with long s-shaped curves)

Type 3 - Curly (hair with well-defined s-shaped curls)

Type 4 - Kinky (hair with tight coils or hair with a less defined curl pattern and more of a zigzag, "z" pattern)

The HTCS is very useful as a **basic** foundation of hair typing knowledge, but it does have its limitations. In reality, a woman will often have more than one type *and* texture of hair on her head throughout her life. It should also be said that all hair is difficult to precisely categorize because of the many different variations from person to person. So, it's not as simple as a particular woman having just one hair type on her head. For example, it's not uncommon to find a black woman that has **both** Type 3 and Type 4 hair. I have a mixture of Type 3 and Type 4 hair.

Because of this complexity in hair typing, other classification systems were created to further break down hair type and texture. The LOIS system is another example of a very popular hair typing system.

I don't want to get overly involved with hair typing because these systems are available for you to research more in-depth at your own discretion. I have simply included Mr. Walker's system because it is easy to understand and despite its limitations, it is still useful because it helps to demonstrate why different types of hair need to be taken care of differently. Curly and kinky hair (Types 3 and 4) will need special care when compared to straight hair. Women with natural Type 4 hair (or a combination of natural Type 4 and Type 3 hair) are often referred to as having "afro-textured" hair. And as far as growing hair, you'll ultimately need to know that afro-textured hair will have three very important characteristics:

Characteristic #1 - It will be finer than other hair types

Characteristic #2 - It will be drier than other hair types

Characteristic #3 - It will be more prone to breakage

Afro-textured hair is finer than other hair types because the surface opening of curly and kinky hair follicles is more oval than circular. Thus, when hair grows from curly or kinky follicles, the hair strand will be a bit flattened due to the shape of the hair follicle. The hair will not be round and uniformly thick like the hair that grows from the l-shaped follicles of straight hair. To get a better mental picture, think of how fettuccine looks when compared to plain spaghetti. Fettuccine represents curly or kinky hair, and spaghetti represents straight hair.

Interestingly enough, when the average person looks at an Afro, they'll tend to think that the hair looks much thicker when compared to straight hair. But, hair strand thickness and perceived hair thickness is not the same thing. An Afro looks thick because the curlier and kinkier nature of the hair allows it to take up more space and appear more voluminous. Although this hair *looks* thick and voluminous, the individual strands can actually be quite thin. In fact, the curlier your hair becomes, the finer it will be. In the case of kinky hair, the strands of hair are actually baby-fine. On top of that, every curl and bend in the hair actually represents a point of weakness and possible breakage. More proof of why women with afro-textured hair need to be very loving with their hair in order for it to grow.

THE SCALP & THE ACID MANTLE

All hair follicles need to have their own supply of blood and glands in order to maintain healthy hair growth. Blood is the communication link between your body and your hair. It carries nutrients and oxygen to your hair follicles so that they can function. The blood vessels that feed hair follicles are located at the base of the follicle. These blood vessels are called the dermal papilla. Though the dermal papilla doesn't actually produce hair (that's the hair follicle's job), the dermal papilla still has the ability to directly influence hair growth and hair loss, as you will soon learn.

Along with the dermal papilla, there is another structure that is important in hair growth. This structure sits near the top of the hair follicle, just beneath the surface of the skin. It is a sac-like structure known as the sebaceous gland. Sebaceous glands produce sebum, an oily substance that coats the skin and hair for protection and natural conditioning.

SEBUM—HAIR'S NATURAL CONDITIONER

Women with afro-textured hair often wonder why our hair tends to be drier than other hair types. The answer is found in sebum, the hair's natural conditioner. Sebum's oily consistency makes it perfect for locking moisture into hair. Moisture (i.e. water) is a vital component to hair. Moisture is what gives hair its elasticity and the ability to bend and not break under manipulation. Moisture is also what keeps your skin soft and supple. When hair or skin lacks moisture, it will become dry.

Moisture is being continually absorbed and lost by our hair. This is why Mother Nature created sebum. Sebum works to seal moisture into our hair and skin. As you already know, oil and water do not mix. When you place oil and water in a glass, the oil will rise to the top and keep the water locked in place below. This is the same thing that happens with sebum. When sebum is released from sebaceous glands, it will form a barrier that locks moisture into the scalp and hair.

In straighter hair types, sebum is able to easily travel down the hair shaft and seal in moisture along the entire length of the hair. This is not the case in afro-textured hair. The bends, coils and curls make it harder for sebum to travel down the hair shaft. In fact, sometimes it may be near impossible for sebum to even make it halfway down the length of a curly or kinky strand of hair. For this reason, curlier and kinkier hair tends to lack a moisture protective shield. As a result, afro-textured hair tends to be drier than straight hair because it is prone to losing moisture more easily.

This is why I mentioned that the water content of hair is one of the key factors that will determine whether afro-textured hair grows to longer lengths. Dryness is a constant issue in afro-textured hair types. However, this problem can be easily combated by increasing the water content of hair through moisturizing. Hair that is properly moisturized will not be dry and break as easily. So, from now on take note that moisturizing your hair is one key thing that you will need to do in order to grow your hair to longer lengths.

SEBUM VERSUS SWEAT

Sometimes, people think of sebum and sweat as the same thing coming from the same gland. But, sebum and sweat are actually two totally different substances that come from two totally different glands. These substances also have separate and distinguishing functions.

Sweat glands produce sweat, which helps to regulate body temperature. Think back to a ridiculously hot, dry summer day. Remember how the sun was beating down and you were drenched in sweat? How did it feel when a nice breeze hit your skin? Felt like heaven, huh? The reason why your body instantly felt cooler was because of sweat. The air hitting your moist skin created a cooling effect. Sweat cools you off and keeps your body from overheating.

Although sweat is used as a thermoregulator, this is not its only function. When mixed with the sebum from sebaceous glands, sweat also helps to form a thin, protective layer on the skin and hair called the *acid mantle*. The acid mantle is a very important barrier that helps to protect our bodies from invading viruses, bacteria, fungus, and other microorganisms. In fact, it is a change in the acid mantle that actually causes dandruff. Dandruff is simply the result of fungal overgrowth on the scalp.

The acid mantle is called such because it has an acidic pH. The term pH (which is an abbreviation for "power of hydrogen") is used to describe the acidity or alkalinity of a solution. The pH scale ranges from the number 0 to 14, with a pH of 7.0 being neutral. Pure water has a neutral pH or a pH of 7.0. Solutions with a pH greater than 7.0 are considered basic (or alkaline), while solutions with a pH lower than 7.0 are acidic. Our hair and skin's acid mantle normally sits at a pH between 4.5 and 5.5, which means our hair and skin is actually more acidic than water.

The acid mantle is a very effective barrier against invading microorganisms, and it also serves to protect the structure of your hair. Any substance that significantly alters the pH of the acid mantle can permanently alter and even degrade the protein structure of hair. This is the case with "lye" and "no-lye" relaxers which can have pH ranges from 10-14.

Each step up or below a number on the pH scale represents a tenfold increase in alkalinity (moving up the scale) or in acidity (moving down the scale). Knowing this, you can now see that relaxers are significantly more alkaline than hair. In fact, a relaxer with a pH of 11 can be up to **one million** times more alkaline than hair.

It is this significant difference in pH that enables relaxers to permanently alter the protein structure of hair, taking hair that was once curly, and making it permanently straight. This change in pH also weakens the hair strand.

Hair is very sensitive to changes in pH, so hair must be pH balanced in order to retain its strength and structural integrity. This is especially the case after any chemical process. Take relaxing hair as an example. If a relaxer is simply washed from the hair without a neutralizing shampoo to bring the pH of hair back down to normal (or as close to normal as possible), hair will actually become brittle and ultimately break. This happens because the drastic change in pH has altered the protein structure of the hair. As a result, relaxers need to be followed up with some sort of neutralizing agent, typically a neutralizing shampoo. The neutralizing shampoo helps to "neutralize" the relaxer effects, restore pH balance and recondition the hair shaft.

Relaxers aren't the only things that can alter the pH of the acid mantle. Chemical processes such as commercial hair coloring, shampoos, conditioners, and many other everyday hair products can also alter the acid mantle. Nowadays, many shampoos and conditioner products are already "pH balanced," meaning that they will not significantly increase or decrease the pH of the acid mantle. But, this is not the case for all commercial products.

Ultimately it is up to you to be aware of the pH of your hair care products; both commercial and homemade. The pH of your hair products can be easily tested by using pH testing strips (i.e. Litmus paper) that can be purchased online or via select pharmacies. The key thing to remember is that you should always attempt to keep the acid mantle of your hair within its normal 4.5 to 5.5 range. Increases and decreases in the pH of the acid mantle can weaken the protein structure of your hair, lead to breakage, and ultimately counteract hair growth.

THE STRUCTURE OF HAIR

A strand of hair consists of three layers:

Cuticle - the outermost layer

Cortex - the middle layer

Medulla - the innermost layer (only present in thick, coarse hair types)

THE CUTICLE

The cuticle is your hair's first line of defense against damage. It is a thin, colorless layer that serves as the protector for the inner layers of hair. If you were to look at a strand of hair under a microscope, the surface of the hair would look scaly, almost resembling the shingles on a rooftop. Under normal, healthy hair conditions the cuticle will be flat and smooth. However, the cuticle layer can slightly lift under certain circumstances. For example, you can raise the cuticle of the hair by:

- Increasing the surface temperature of the hair with direct heat.

- Increasing the pH of the acid mantle.

When the cuticle is raised, the interior of the hair strand will be more exposed and vulnerable to damage and moisture loss. While raising the cuticle may always seem like a bad thing, it can be beneficial under certain conditions. For example, when conditioning hair, you may want to slightly raise the cuticle to allow deeper penetration of conditioner into the inner layers of your hair. This is why heat is sometimes used when deep conditioning hair. The heat causes the cuticle to rise, resulting in increased conditioner penetration and a more enhanced moisturizing effect. After deep conditioning with heat, it is also wise to rinse your hair with cool or cold water. You want to do this because the change in temperature will cause the cuticle to lower again. Remember, flat cuticles protect the inner structures of the hair.

Though the cuticle is in place to protect, it is important to note that the cuticle of your hair does not function like a door on a hinge. Your cuticle doesn't just swing open and shut. The cuticle is actually fragile and will wear down or chip away with repetitious movement. Keep this in mind when taking care of your hair. You will learn more about the specific sources of cuticle damage later on.

In addition to serving as a source of protection, the cuticle layer also gives hair its shine or sheen. In all hair types, flat cuticles will reflect a certain degree of light. In the case of straight hair, light is reflected easily and almost perfectly off of the surface of the hair, giving hair an appearance of shine. In the case of curlier/kinkier hair, light reflection becomes a bit less perfect due to the bends, twists and twirls in the hair strand. As a result, this type of hair will produce smaller reflections of light known as sheen. Shine and sheen are simply variable degrees of the same thing- the reflection of light. And though afro-textured hair may not look as shiny as straight hair, this does not mean it is any less healthy. An intact cuticle is a great determinant of hair's health, not its high degree of shine.

THE CORTEX

The cortex is the middle and thickest layer of the hair shaft. It makes up the bulk of your hair's structure and it's where most of your hair's protein and moisture reside. The cortex also determines other unique characteristics of your hair, such as its color. Most importantly, the cortex determines your hair's strength and elasticity. Strength and elasticity are also very important factors that will determine if hair will grow to longer lengths.

So what is it about the cortex that gives hair its strength?

The cortex's protein structure is held together by two major types of bonds: physical bonds and chemical bonds. Overall, both types of bonds are working to reinforce the strength of the hair shaft. Physical bonds include hydrogen bonds and salt bonds. These bonds are weaker, more flexible and can be easily broken and reformed by physical processes like exposure to water and heat. The effects of breaking physical bonds are temporary and once bonds reconfigure, hair will be returned to its original state, be it curly or straight. Flat ironing and wet-setting hair are two examples of physical processes that can break and reform physical bonds.

In addition to physical bonds, the cortex's protein structure is also held together by chemical bonds. These bonds are significantly stronger than physical bonds. Disulfide bonds and peptide bonds are the chemical bonds in hair. These types of bonds can only be broken by stronger chemical processes. The breaking of chemical bonds results in a permanent change in the protein structure of hair. Furthermore, once chemical bonds are broken, they cannot be reformed to their original state. Thus, hair will be weaker than before. Relaxers and permanent dyes are common chemical processes that can break the chemical bonds in hair.

The structure and bonding configuration of the cortex is pretty intricate. In fact, many people think of a strand of hair as one single thing, but a single strand of hair is actually many smaller components woven together. As stated earlier, hair is made primarily of protein. The building blocks of protein are tiny structures called amino acids. If you were to take a series of amino acids and bond them together, they would form a structure called a polypeptide chain. The polypeptide chain looks somewhat like pearls on a string. Several polypeptide chains will crosslink and form helixes, which look like spiral ladders. Theses helixes will also crosslink to form threadlike fibers that twist around each other to make larger bundles called microfibrils. Many microfibrils will then twist around each other to form macrofibrils. Finally, macrofibrils will intertwine to form fibrils. The bonding and intertwining of the amino acids, polypeptide chains, microfibrils, macrofibrils, and fibrils is what forms and reinforces the strength of the hair. Ultimately, it is the physical and chemical bonds that allow all these components to come together as one strand of hair.

Now that you've learned what gives hair its strength, it's time to learn what gives hair its elasticity.

The cortex is the layer that provides strength, and it is also the layer that absorbs water. Water is what gives hair its ability to bend and stretch under manipulation. This ability to bend and stretch is known as *elasticity*. Water, which is commonly referred to as the "ultimate moisturizer," is what helps to break physical bonds and soften the hardened protein structure of hair. Without adequate moisture, the protein structure of hair will become more dry and rigid. This type of hair lacks elasticity and will break. So once again, hair not only needs a strong protein structure, it also needs moisture in order to grow to longer lengths.

PROTEIN & MOISTURE- BALANCING FOR GROWTH

Balancing protein and moisture becomes very important when attempting to grow hair to longer lengths. This is because protein and moisture will determine your hair's strength and elasticity. Life and growth is about balance- and your hair is no different. So you will need to pay very close attention to maintaining your hair's protein and moisture balance. This sounds straightforward, but achieving balance is not as simple as constantly feeding your hair moisture and protein. Too much of one or the other will cause imbalance and weaken your hair. For example, too much moisture can make your hair very soft and gummy. Too much protein can dry your hair and make it prone to breakage. Overall, you'll need to be mindful of how much protein and moisture you give your hair on a regular basis. If hair becomes weakened from an imbalance, it will be a lot harder to grow because it will break under the normal stresses of regular maintenance.

How can you check for and maintain protein and moisture balance? The easiest way to tell if your hair has a proper balance of protein and moisture is to do a wet strand test. You can do this by taking a wet strand of hair, stretching it, and observing how it reacts.

When stretched, balanced hair will feel strong. It will stretch to a certain degree, and not immediately break. On the other hand, hair that lacks moisture will not feel strong. It will feel brittle, straw-like, and will almost immediately pop when stretched. Most afro-textured hair will lack moisture. It's just a common characteristic within our hair type. Some women with afro-textured hair may notice that their hair lacks protein instead of moisture. When these women pull their hair it may stretch and stretch like Laffy Taffy. This is hair that is over-moisturized or lacks protein. You don't tend to see this condition too often with afro-textured hair, but it can happen and it is a sign that hair is imbalanced.

Achieving and maintaining protein and moisture balance is not an exact science. Still women usually want very specific guidelines on protein and moisture balancing. I must emphasize that every head of hair is different and you'll just need to pay close attention to your hair and exercise good judgment. A good rule of thumb is to moisturize more than you use protein. This is because it's very easy to give afro-textured hair too much protein. Rarely do you have cases where afro-textured hair is over-moisturized. If you want more specific directions then this, I'd recommend that you moisturize daily, and use protein treatments once every six to eight weeks. This is the regimen I follow and many women follow regimens similar to this. It's pretty simple, and it's been quite effective in helping me achieve and maintain a protein and moisture balance for my afro-textured hair.

THE CYCLES OF HAIR GROWTH

Hair grows in a cycle of three phases: a growth phase (anagen), a transition phase (catagen) and a resting phase (telogen).

ANAGEN- THE GROWTH PHASE

- Hair follicles produce hair at approximately ½ inch (or 1.25 cm) per month

- Normally, up to 90% of hair follicles are in the anagen phase at any given time

- On average, this phase lasts between 2-8 years

- As we age, the duration of the anagen phase begins to shorten

CATAGEN- THE TRANSITION PHASE

- Approximately 2-3% of hair follicles are in a transitional phase at any given time

- During this phase, a club hair (a transparent bulb) begins to form at the lower portion of the hair shaft in contact with the hair follicle

- The formation of club hair cuts off the blood supply from the dermal papilla and signals the end of the active growth phase of a hair

- Phase lasts between 2-4 weeks

TELOGEN- THE RESTING PHASE

- Approximately 10% to 15% of hair follicles are in the resting phase at any given time

- During this phase, the formation of the club hair becomes complete and the hair is in a fully rested state preparing to be shed

There is also a seldom-acknowledged fourth phase of the hair cycle known as exogen. This phase is actually independent of the telogen phase. The exogen phase is also referred to as the shedding phase. During the exogen phase, hair is actually shed. After hair is shed, a new hair growth cycle begins with anagen.

HAIR GROWTH FACTORS

There are five major factors that influence hair growth: genetics, hormones, nutrition, exercise and stress.

GENETICS

Since they are not under our control, I will not take much time discussing the role of genetics in hair growth. Still, you should know that your genes are responsible for influencing many factors when it comes to your hair and hair growth. Your genes will determine things like your hair color, the shape of your hair follicles, the number of hair follicles on your head (which will never change no matter how old you get) as well as your rate of hair growth.

HORMONES

Think of hormones as tiny little messengers traveling all through your body. A hormone is a chemical released by cells. When a hormone is released, it will enter a blood vessel and navigate the body via the bloodstream. Your blood and blood vessels function as a hormone's transportation system. Once released, a hormone has the ability to travel from one part of your body to another, influencing target cells in any other part of the body.

A hormone interacts with a target cell via receptor sites on that specific cell. Different cells in our bodies have different receptor sites for different hormones. Hormones can only affect cells that carry a designated receptor site. So, when a hormone finds its receptor cell, it has found the lock for its designated key. The key turns and a chain of events are set into motion that will tell the cell what to do. Basically, hormones allow cells to talk to and influence each other. We wouldn't be able to carry out our body's vital functions without hormones. Many living things use hormones, even plants!

In women, there are several hormones that influence hair growth. A few of these hormones are cortisol, estrogen, progesterone, testosterone and thyroid hormone. Yes ladies, just like the fellas, our bodies also produce testosterone.

Our ovaries produce estrogen, progesterone and testosterone. Our adrenal glands (small glands that sit on top of our kidneys) produce the hormones cortisol, estrogen, and testosterone. Last, but not least, our thyroid gland produces thyroid hormone.

All of these hormones (in addition to other factors) affect hair growth and the hair growth cycle, either by increasing hair growth, decreasing hair growth, or stopping it altogether. Hormones are also influenced by many factors, including age, pregnancy, menopause, stress, and even by the foods and medications that we put into our body.

Hormones can be a very complicated topic, but I wanted to share one simple example of how hormones influence hair growth. Let's take a look closer look at what happens during pregnancy.

Pregnancy is actually a very interesting time for hormonal change. Almost all pregnant women will experience an increased rate in hair growth during pregnancy, often resulting in thicker and longer hair. Many women assume that this change in hair growth is due to prenatal vitamins, but that's not the case. Prenatal vitamins do provide an abundance of nutrients for healthy hair growth, but during pregnancy the increased rate of hair growth is due to hormonal fluctuations, not vitamins. During pregnancy there are certain hormonal changes that help a Mommy-to-be's body adjust to the new life growing inside of her. These hormonal changes are necessary to carry a pregnancy to term. So, the hormones are concerned with keeping Mommy and baby healthy, not with whether Mommy has a gorgeous head of hair. One of these hormones is estrogen. During pregnancy, hair growth is simply a side effect of higher levels of estrogen that coincidentally lock hair follicles in the anagen and catagen phase.

Shortly after a mother gives birth, her hormone levels will fluctuate once again. Now that she's no longer pregnant, her body will signal a hormone readjustment and the side effect of readjustment will be hair shedding. In fact, the shedding can be quite extensive, but thankfully temporary. This temporary shedding is commonly known as postpartum shedding, but the medical term is actually *telogen effluvium* or *postpartum alopecia*.

Postpartum shedding can be a scary experience, but fortunately it's just a temporary effect of hormone readjustment. The shedding will eventually stop and normal hair growth will resume. So don't worry Mommy-to-be's; you will have to sacrifice sleep while tending to your bundles of joy, but you won't have to sacrifice all the hairs on your head. You'll still be a hot momma- with a full head of hair!

NUTRITION

Hair consists of approximately 91% protein which comes directly from our diet. When we eat certain foods, our digestive system works to break this food down to its most basic nutrients (e.g. amino acids, vitamins and minerals). These smaller nutrients are then sent to all the other cells in our body, where tiny cells in hair follicles use these building blocks to produce hair.

Nutrition and hair growth is actually quite straightforward. But there's a catch: It's not as simple as eating food and expecting hair to grow in healthy and strong. In fact, your body has a very specific hierarchy that it follows when determining which cells and body parts will receive nutrients first. Unfortunately, your hair and nails are not high on the priority list.

Think of it this way: your body is made of millions of cells. All of these cells need nutrients to grow and function. Your body is designed to maintain function and growth in the worst possible case scenario- starvation. In cases of starvation or poor nutrition, certain cells are automatically designated to receive nutrients first. This will leave other cells to fend for themselves.

Take your brain for example. It is made up of countless cells that are set to receive a massive amount of nutrients from the foods you eat. Your brain is the most important organ in your body. Your brain controls countless body functions. Every breath you take, every beat of your heart, and even how well you comprehend the words on this page are determined by brain function. Your brain helps you do everything! You wouldn't be able to do much without it.

That being understood, now think about how smart it would be for your body to direct nutrients to your hair follicle cells before your brain cells. Not very smart! Yes, you'd have a great head of hair, but all at the risk of depriving the very organ that keeps you alive. Not a good look.

In fact, there are many more organs and cells that maintain vital body functions and thus, take priority over your hair follicle cells. Your heart cells, kidney cells, liver cells, and lung cells are just a few. This is precisely why a full and healthy diet is always emphasized for hair growth. If you want your hair cells to get the nutrients that they need to produce hair at maximum potential, you'll need to provide *all* of your body's cells with an abundance of nutrients.

EXERCISE

Are you the type of person that steers clear of exercise because you don't want to mess up your hair? I hate to break it to you, but skipping exercise may be doing your hair more harm than good. Did you know that exercise actually stimulates hair growth?

Here are a few ways exercise stimulates hair growth:

- Exercise helps regulate the glands which produce the hormones that will stimulate hair follicles

- Exercise improves blood flow and nutrient delivery to the dermal papilla, which will stimulate hair follicles

- Exercise boosts your metabolism, which will accelerate the rate at which your hair follicles produce hair

- Exercise reduces the release of cortisol (the "stress hormone"), which is responsible for pushing hair into the telogen phase

For the ladies who regularly skip exercise to keep their hair looking nice, you may want to reconsider your whole plan of action. Hair growth and exercise actually go hand in hand. Furthermore, it goes without saying that one should always strive to live a healthy lifestyle. Regular exercise is a part of that, regardless of whether you want to grow hair longer or not.

I once had to speak with a young black patient about her weight and general health. She was an 18 year old girl with a BMI (body mass index) of 29, meaning she was severely overweight. She also had symptoms of metabolic syndrome- a very serious condition where an individual exhibits signs/symptoms of high blood sugar, high cholesterol, high blood pressure and increased weight. Metabolic syndrome is a very serious condition that predisposes individuals to developing other deadly conditions like coronary artery disease, stroke, and Type 2 diabetes.

I explained the seriousness of her condition, while recommending exercise and other lifestyle changes that would help her to lose weight. My patient seemed genuinely concerned about her overall health, but when asked about what steps she planned to take to tackle her weight issues, she expressed uncertainty about how she would be able to exercise regularly. She was willing to change her eating habits, but she was a bit more resistant to exercising. When I asked why, she basically explained that she didn't like to sweat because it messed up her hair.

I wish I could say I haven't encountered other black women who said the same thing when confronted with serious weight and health issues, but that wouldn't be the truth. It's important to note that black women aren't the only race of women that make certain lifestyle choices that adversely affect our health. We aren't the only race of women that worry about our hair either. But, it is a fact that women within the black community are more likely to die from conditions that are completely avoided through regular exercise.

In fact, many of the common yet serious health issues that we see today result from lack of exercise. Potentially fatal conditions like heart disease (the number one killer of all women) and Type 2 diabetes are both examples of conditions that are preventable and even curable with diet and exercise.

I know many women that skip the gym because of their hair. It's unfortunate, because they're basically jeopardizing their overall health to "save" their hair. But what good is nice hair when you're suffering from diabetes or lying in a coffin? It's not a good look when you put your hair over health. So don't skimp on exercise. You'll do your health and hair better service in the long run.

STRESS

Stress is a HUGE factor in hair growth, which is why I wanted to leave it for last. Stress is a major player in hair growth because it can affect the previous four factors I mentioned. Stress can affect your hormones. Stress can affect what and how often you eat. It can also influence whether or not you want to exercise. Stress can even affect your genes!

We all know that stress can be very unpleasant, as well as unavoidable. Stress is just a natural part of life and fortunately our bodies are hard-wired to react to stress in ways that are meant to protect us. This hardwiring exists from back in the days when we were fighting saber-toothed tigers and running from dinosaurs. OK, maybe that's a bit of an exaggeration but suffice to say, our bodies have evolved to have a specific response to threats (or stress). This response is called the *fight or flight response.*

At times when you're feeling anxiety or pressure from things like a hectic work schedule, a nagging family member, or even a barking dog, your body will recognize this stress as a threat and activate the fight or flight response. The fight or flight response is like an alarm system that goes off and signals your adrenal glands to release the stress hormone cortisol, as well as the hormone adrenaline. These hormones make you want to get up and get moving! Without such a response we wouldn't know when or how to respond to stress or danger. This hormonal response is in place to protect us and is essential for survival. However, this is also a system that should not remain activated for long periods of time. This is because prolonged exposure to adrenaline and cortisol can have significant negative effects and cause a general decline in health. Prolonged cortisol exposure can also adversely affect hair growth. In fact, hair loss can be a symptom of chronic stress.

Cortisol is a hormone that has the ability to affect many of the other hormones that affect hair growth. It can also push the hair cycle into the telogen phase, which means cortisol can trigger the premature and even massive shedding of hair. In fact, chronic stress and hair loss can function as a vicious cycle that feeds on itself. This is how it happens: When you're under stress, you will lose some hair. When you see hair falling out you'll start to worry some more about your hair loss. When you worry some more, you'll get more stressed out and cortisol will remain elevated. Then you'll lose more hair. It's a snowball effect.

This is why it's essential to positively manage stress in order to maintain healthy hair growth. Stress, big or small, will always be a part of your life. But, if you are able to handle stress effectively by doing things like exercise, praying, meditation, getting massages and even aromatherapy, cortisol will remained balanced and you will continue to enjoy a healthy head of hair.

TAKE HOME POINTS

Afro-textured hair has 3 key characteristics that will affect its growth potential:

1. It will be finer than other hair types

2. It will be drier than other hair types

3. It will be more prone to breakage

Sebum functions as a natural conditioner and locks moisture into hair. It is the poor distribution of sebum along the hair shaft of afro-textured hair that contributes to its dryness.

The acid mantle serves as a barrier against invading microorganisms and also works to protect the protein structure of hair. Any substance that alters the pH of the acid mantle can permanently alter and even degrade the protein structure of hair.

The cortex of the hair provides strength through its protein structure and elasticity through its water content.

The balance of protein and moisture is essential to growing hair to longer lengths. A good rule of thumb is to moisturize afro-textured hair daily and use protein treatments every six to eight weeks.

Hair grows in a cycle of three phases: a growth phase (anagen), a transition phase (catagen) and a resting phase (telogen). There is also the lesser acknowledged phase of shedding (exogen).

The five major factors that influence hair growth are genetics, hormones, nutrition, exercise and stress.

CHAPTER 4
BASICS OF HAIR DAMAGE

Growing hair to longer lengths is about striking a balance where your hair growth far surpasses hair damage and breakage. Basically, growing longer hair is about loving your hair more than you are damaging it. The concept is actually pretty simple, but for some women the road to longer hair is a bit difficult. Why does this happen? Why do some women have a hard time achieving length, while others don't? The answer will always lay in how well you treat your hair.

Unfortunately, many of us think we can chronically neglect and damage our hair without affecting growth. We tend to think this because our hair seems so resilient. We can smash it against our pillows when we lay our heads to rest at night. We can get up in the morning and wash it, pull it, tie it, and sometimes even fry it and dye it. We manhandle our hair. We take our hair for granted. We don't think too much about loving our hair and protecting it. Then, after all this abuse we still expect our hair to grow longer if we throw an occasional deep conditioner or protein treatment on it. Unfortunately, that's just not the way it works.

No matter how resilient or strong your hair may *appear* to be, the truth is that your hair is actually quite delicate. It is as delicate as a silk blouse. This type of garment is made of many fibers - just like our hair. Remember those microfibrils, macrofibrils and fibrils that form the cortex? These individual fibrils (or fibers) are woven together to form a strand of hair, much like individual fibers of material that are woven together to form a silk blouse. The fibers come together to form something beautiful and stronger than one single strand of material.

You should always think of handling your hair as if you were handling a silk blouse. You wouldn't just throw a silk blouse in the wash and dump any type of detergent on it. You wouldn't use a ton of heat to dry or iron it either. You wouldn't do any of these things because it would ruin the delicate material. When you want to keep a precious garment looking nice for as long as possible, you're taught to treat it with the utmost care. This is how you should also treat your hair.

HAIR TYPE & DAMAGE POTENTIAL

While all hair should be treated with the utmost care, women with afro-textured hair need to be especially mindful of how they handle their hair. Curlier and kinkier hair, by its very nature, is more delicate and finer than straight hair. So, in order to gain length, your hair must be regularly treated with love.

Unfortunately, there are factors every day that are working to gradually damage your hair by stripping away the cuticle (your hair's first line of defense). There are also factors working to rob your hair of moisture. If you're not mindful about protecting your hair, the effects of damage will accumulate and you'll end up with hair that's dry, dull, breaking, and in some cases even falling out from the root.

This is why it's best to learn about the common sources of hair damage as well as the best ways to avoid them. Four common causes of hair damage include chemical damage, physical damage, environmental damage and damage from poor nutrition.

CHEMICAL DAMAGE

Chemically processing your hair will always cause damage. This means that chemical processes like relaxers, texturizers (which are simply mild relaxers), other chemical hair straighteners (i.e. the Brazilian Keratin treatment), and many commercial hair dyes, will all damage hair to varying degrees. Chemical processing will permanently alter the hair shaft by penetrating the cuticle layer of the hair and breaking protein bonds in the cortex. Contrary to popular belief, no matter how "gentle" a manufacturer or stylist claims a chemical process is, the truth is that your hair will experience some degree of damage from it. Furthermore, using multiple chemical processes will have an even more damaging effect on hair, making it significantly weaker than before.

PHYSICAL DAMAGE

Physical damage occurs when hair is manipulated in any way. Whenever you wash, comb, brush, roller-set, flat iron, blow dry, or simply handle your hair, it will require some degree of hair manipulation. No matter how gentle you are being to your hair, manipulation will always result in some degree of hair damage. The extent of the damage will vary depending on the amount of physical force you use to manipulate your hair. Physical damage can happen with just about anything that requires moving your hair, but there are four very common causes of physical hair damage that you should look out for: combs/brushes, heat styling, hygral fatigue and commercial hair products.

Combs & Brushes

Many women use combs and brushes for regular hair grooming but what would you think if I told you that your comb and brush could be literally tearing your hair apart? Without a doubt, combs and brushes can wreak havoc on the cuticles of your hair. Furthermore, when the bristles of brushes and teeth of combs make direct contact with the scalp, they also have the ability to pull hair straight out from the follicle. I honestly cringe every time I see a woman using a comb to rip through her tangles or when

I see a woman using a brush to "massage" her scalp. Many women with afro-textured hair rely on combs and brushes for grooming, and unfortunately these types of hair tools can do tremendously more harm than good.

Heat Styling

There are many women like myself who grew up believing that heat styling is perfectly harmless. I remember flat-ironing, curling and blow-drying without much thought of the damage it was doing to my hair. I know better now. Heat styling is definitely not as harmless as we'd like to think.

Heat is able to shape hair because it breaks protein bonds. In addition, heat, even at low settings, has the ability to damage the cuticle. At higher temperatures, heat can even melt the protein structure of the hair. Besides all of that, heat can literally boil moisture right out of the hair shaft and cause a condition known as *bubble hair*. Bubble hair occurs when the moisture in hair is heated, turns to steam, evaporates, and bubbles the hair. The bubbling effect damages the internal structure of the hair shaft and can even rupture the cortex and cuticle layer.

The cuticle protects your hair. The protein structure of the cortex gives your hair strength. Moisture gives your hair elasticity. Your hair needs a healthy cuticle, an intact protein structure, and a good degree of moisture to maintain its integrity. Without all of these factors working together to reinforce strength and elasticity, your hair will break, even with gentle manipulation.

The take home point is that heat is not harmless. To the contrary, it can be very damaging. When you use things like flat-irons and blow dryers, you break bonds, destroy your cuticle, leech moisture right out of your hair, and ultimately dry your hair out. This all spells trouble for hair in general, but especially for afro-textured hair, since this type of hair is already quite delicate and already prone to dryness.

Hygral Fatigue

Hygral fatigue is a type of damage that occurs when the hair shaft is repeatedly stressed by the effects of wetting and drying. This is how the damage happens: when you wet your hair, moisture will be absorbed into the inner structure of the hair. The cuticle will slightly rise as the hair shaft swells from moisture entering the cortex. This puts tension on the hair shaft. When the hair shaft dries, it will begin to contract back to normal size. The contraction can be very rapid and very stressful to the structure of the hair. This is especially the case when heat is used to quickly dry hair.

Hygral fatigue, in a sense, causes damage to the hair shaft from the inside out. After enough times of your cuticle raising and flattening, and your hair expanding and contracting, the hair shaft will become stressed and damaged. In some cases, the hair shaft may even be stretched to the point of literally "popping" in certain areas. If that explanation was a bit difficult to visualize, think of what happens when you squeeze yourself into a cute baby t-shirt that's just a wee bit too tight. *We've all done it, ladies.* When you squeeze yourself in, you put stress on the shirt's material and the seams. The t-shirt will stretch to accommodate you, but you end up stretching out the material more than it was meant to stretch. After enough washes and wears, you end up with a shirt that's permanently stretched to a slightly larger size. You may even end up with a t-shirt that has a few popped seams. This is exactly what happens to your hair when it becomes damaged by hygral fatigue.

Your hair readily absorbs water, just like a t-shirt will absorb water. After your hair stretches and shrinks enough times, you'll end up with hair that has a more stretched or "ballooned" structure. The cuticle will become damaged, the internal structure of the hair will become damaged, and some areas of the hair may balloon to the point of rupture or tearing. Remember, your hair is a delicate fiber. Just like the fibers that make up your t-shirt. Hygral fatigue can affect all hair types, not just afro-textured hair, and hygral fatigue is especially an issue with highly porous hair.

Porosity refers to the hair's ability (or inability) to absorb water or chemicals into the cortex. All hair is naturally porous and will absorb some degree of water and certain types of chemicals. Afro-textured hair tends to be on the low end of porosity. So, my hair will not accept moisture or chemicals as readily as say, a person with Type 1 hair. For afro-textured hair to become highly porous it must have cuticles that are defective *and* it must also have a protein structure that lacks some degree of integrity. In the simplest terms, highly porous afro-textured hair is sign that hair has been damaged.

You will typically encounter highly porous hair in cases where hair has been processed with chemicals or damaged from other sources such as heat. Ideally, hair should maintain some degree of porosity so that it can readily accept moisture. But, afro-textured hair should not be highly porous because this means that moisture will move too easily in and out of its structure. When hair becomes too porous, it has the ability to accept too much moisture. It also has the ability to lose too much moisture. In the case of highly porous hair, more moisture will be lost than accepted. This is why women with this hair condition tend to complain about hair that's constantly dry regardless of how much they moisturize.

Commercial Hair Products
Commercial products themselves are not the cause of physical damage. It's the ingredients in certain commercial hair products that can damage hair. One example is sodium laureth sulfate (SLS), an ingredient found in most commercial shampoos.

Sulfates are strong cleansing agents that are extremely drying to hair. Commonly used sulfates are sodium lauryl sulfate, ammonium laureth sulfate and sodium laureth sulfate. These are the agents that give shampoos (and other cleansers) their sudsy and foaming ability. Besides the majority of shampoos, you can also find sulfates in body washes, laundry detergent, and even oven cleaner. Many of us have been conditioned to love and even expect the wonderful lather and bubbles that come from our commercial shampoos. But, this bubbly goodness is actually quite damaging to hair. This is because sulfates are powerful degreasers. When used on things like grimy ovens, sulfates work wonderfully. But when used on hair, sulfates will literally strip all oils, including sebum. Thus, using most types of commercial shampoos will actually lead to hair that is drier and more prone to breakage.

Product overload is another example of how commercial ingredients can damage hair. This happens because certain agents in products will bind very tightly to hair. When these agents are allowed to sit on the hair and scalp for extended periods of time, they will work to block moisture from entering the hair. These agents can also accumulate on the scalp and even stifle the hair follicle. One agent that can do this is silicone, a very common ingredient in commercial conditioners.

Silicone works by coating the hair shaft and forming a seal around the cuticle. Silicone gives hair incredible shine and also works great for detangling by giving hair "slip." Slip is best described as a wet, sea-weedy feeling that helps the hair shafts to move past each other without much friction. Women tend to love the effect of silicones on their hair, and I don't know many women who wouldn't like shinier and more manageable hair. But while silicones can be great ingredients in commercial products, there are certain types of silicones that can buildup on hair and cause damage.

There are many different types of silicones, some being stronger than others. The stronger silicones are not water-soluble and have the ability to form a coat on the hair shaft that is impenetrable to water. This coat will not only prevent moisture from getting out of the hair, it will also prevent moisture from getting in. It is the stronger silicones that have the ability to eventually buildup on hair and cause dryness. I will give more information on silicones in a later chapter, but the key thing to remember here is that you need to be mindful of the ingredients in your commercial hair products. If not, hair damage from product buildup will become an issue.

ENVIRONMENTAL DAMAGE

Environmental damage is the direct result of exposing hair to the elements. Some causes of environmental damage are sun exposure (UV ray exposure), temperature extremes (i.e. cold, dry air), air pollutants, beach water, chlorine water and, most commonly, hard water from your showerhead.

According to the United States Geological Survey, over 80% of US homes have hard water. Hard water is simply water that contains a high amount of dissolved minerals like calcium and magnesium. Hard water is not a big deal per se, but for those who don't have water softeners or water filters, hard water can become a problem when minerals build-up on the hair shaft and the scalp. Hard water mineral buildup will form a coat that makes cleansing, moisturizing and conditioning more difficult. For example, when calcium deposits build on the hair shaft, it can form a film that binds tightly to agents in shampoos, conditioners and other styling products. When these agents bind to calcium, hair will become dull and weighed down due to mineral and product buildup. The mineral and product buildup on the hair will also block out moisture. This leads to dryness and breakage. Calcium or other minerals can also accumulate on the scalp causing irritation and flaking, similar to dandruff.

DAMAGE FROM POOR NUTRITION

Once again, I'm going to touch on nutrition because it's constantly underestimated in its importance for hair growth. Hair comes from the inside out. So hair is a reflection of your overall nutritional state. If your body does not get an abundance of nutrients – most especially protein – your hair follicle cells will not get all the building blocks that they need to produce hair. When your hair follicles get a short supply of building blocks, they may still produce hair, but it will be hair that is structurally weaker. Ultimately, a poor diet will result in hair that is defective before it even emerges from your scalp. Once this defective hair is exposed to sources of damage, it will be more likely to break because its structural integrity is defective.

Poor nutrition can even affect the health of your scalp. Your scalp is simply skin; just like the skin on your face or the rest of your body. And can you guess what your skin is primarily made of? If you said "protein," you'd be right! Here's another fun fact: Your skin is actually the largest organ of your body, and just like hair, the overall health and appearance of your skin will be a direct reflection of your overall protein intake. I just wanted to quickly touch on the importance of protein intake now because it is the most important nutrient to growing healthy, strong hair while also maintaining healthy skin and a healthy scalp. Later on, we'll talk more in-depth about protein and other important nutrients for healthy hair growth. Suffice to say, for now I want you to just remember that if you want to grow the *healthiest and strongest hair possible*, you must do all you can to maintain a healthy, balanced and protein-rich diet.

SIGNS OF HAIR DAMAGE

Hair that's damaged will have a certain look and a certain feel. Since the cuticle layer of the hair is the first line of defense, damaged hair will always have damaged cuticles. As a result, damaged cuticles will ultimately lead to hair that has one or more of these physical characteristics: dullness, dryness, split ends, increased tangles, frizziness, increased porosity and….. BREAKAGE!

REPAIRING HAIR DAMAGE

The unfortunate thing about hair damage is that once it's done, it's done. Once hair is damaged, it cannot be repaired to its original strength and integrity, no matter how much moisture, product or protein you throw on it. The only way to completely rid hair of damage is to cut off the part that's damaged.

If you keep damaging your hair, you will experience increased breakage. If you experience increased breakage, you'll have to cut your hair often. This type of scenario is completely counterproductive to growth. This is why you need to fully understand the methods and consequences of hair damage.

You won't achieve length if you keep damaging your hair. Women understand this concept, but sometimes find it hard to align their hair practices with what they know. Maybe you have found yourself in a cycle of dysfunction with your hair. You want longer hair, but you just can't achieve it. Why? It's most likely because you're damaging your hair in some way. It can be very frustrating when you want longer hair, but just can't seem to get past a certain length. I've been there, and it's not fun at all.

In your journey to longer and healthy hair, you must always remember that your hair's potential will be a reflection of how well you treat it and how much you avoid sources of damage. In order for hair to gain length, you must give your hair every fighting chance to grow faster than it breaks. Your hair's growth potential is really in your hands. It's totally up to you whether you will have hair that's healthy and longer, or hair that's unhealthy and breaking. Make your choice, and then do what you have to do to achieve your goal.

TAKE HOME POINTS

The cuticle is your hair's first line of defense.

Four common causes of hair damage include chemical damage, physical damage, environmental damage and damage from poor nutrition.

Eat a balanced, protein-rich diet to maintain a healthy scalp and to also grow your healthiest and strongest hair.

Chemically processing your hair will always cause damage because it permanently alters the hair shaft by penetrating the cuticle layer of the hair and breaking protein bonds in the cortex.

Manipulating your hair in any way will cause variable degrees of damage. The gentler and less frequent you are with manipulation, the less damage will result.

Common signs of hair damage are: dullness, dryness, split ends, increased tangling, frizziness, increased porosity and breakage.

The only way to completely rid hair of damage is to cut off the part that's damaged. No product can restore hair to its original state once damage has been done.

CHAPTER 5
LIFESTYLE PRINCIPLES FOR HEALTHY HAIR GROWTH

Many women ask what I do for my hair, especially what products I use. The thing is, I don't think of my hair's growth and health only in terms of what products I use. Instead, I think of my hair as a reflection of the type of lifestyle that I lead.

I am a woman that strongly advocates approaching hair care from a holistic standpoint, and the reason why is because I know that healthy hair, and longer hair, can only be achieved by first maintaining a healthy lifestyle. So when it comes to growing healthy (and even longer) hair you need to focus on the bigger picture. You need to focus on nutrition (most especially!), exercise, and even stress management for hair growth. And yes, you should also use quality hair products, but most important of all you need to focus on your health first and foremost because healthy hair starts from the inside.

This is why I strive to practice a healthy lifestyle which involves maintaining a healthy diet and a regular exercise regimen, as well as other ways to achieve physical, emotional, and spiritual well-being. Bottom line, when my health is on point, it reflects in my appearance and my hair. Now this isn't to say that I live the "perfect lifestyle" – because I don't by any stretch of the imagination! And sometimes I do fall short of my healthy living goals. Even still, I want to drive home the point that once I gained an understanding that my hair was a reflection of my health, I began treating my hair (and my body) better than I had treated it my entire life. And ultimately, once I got my health together, it was then that my hair began to grow healthier and stronger. This is why I tell women to be extra loving with their hair. I also tell women to approach their hair from a holistic standpoint and make their best effort to follow these 10 lifestyle principles for healthy hair growth.

1. EAT A BALANCED, PROTEIN-RICH DIET

A balanced, protein-rich diet should include whole foods like meat, seafood eggs, fresh vegetables, fresh fruits, nuts, legumes, dairy products, healthy fats and oils, fresh herbs, and spices like pepper which enhance digestion and boost metabolism. You should vary the foods you eat from day to day and eat from a wide variety of fresh foods. You should also drink fresh water daily. The American diet tends to rely heavily on carbonated, caffeinated and sugar-filled drinks. While these types of drinks may taste good, they can also cause dehydration and internal imbalances that can adversely affect your health and your hair.

2. PRACTICE POSITIVE & MINDFUL EATING

When and *how* you eat is just as important as *what* you eat. Mindful eating involves adopting healthy eating habits to promote absorption of nutrients that are important for hair growth. When eating mindfully, you should only eat when hungry and avoid eating when under stress. This means you should avoid "emotional eating" and frequently eating on the go. Food is not just tied to your physical wellbeing; it's also intricately tied to your emotional and spiritual wellbeing. If you're rushed or stressed when you prepare and eat your meal, your body's hormones and digestive system will react negatively. This negativity will then manifest itself in your overall health and your hair. On the contrary, when you practice positive and mindful eating, you will facilitate calm, balance, and enhance your body's ability to take in and positively utilize the nutrients from your food.

3. USE VITAMINS & SUPPLEMENTS

Many women like to use nutritional supplements for hair growth, and I think that's a very smart idea, especially when you consider factors like our less than healthy eating habits, as well as the fact that many of today's foods are in fact less *nutritious* than they were 50 or even 25 years ago due to factors like chemical exposure and soil depletion. Bottom line, we don't live in a perfect world and many of us are not getting enough nutrients from the foods we eat. In addition to that, many of us also slack off on our diets, which mean we're not getting enough of the key nutrients to maximize our hair growth potential. This is why I strongly advocate the **daily** use of high-quality vitamins and nutritional supplements in order to achieve and maintain a healthy, balanced diet, which will then directly lead to healthy hair growth as well as a healthy body overall. In fact, one of my most popular nutritional supplements, *Beauty&Body Protein* (aka *B&B Protein*), is specifically formulated for healthy hair growth as well as healthy weight management, and I have many clients and customers that love using *Beauty&Body Protein* to make post-workout and yummy hair growth smoothies. In chapter 6, *Nutrition and Hair Growth*, I'll get into greater detail about the important role healthy eating plays in hair growth, and in that same chapter I'll also share one of my favorite *B&B Protein Green Smoothie* recipes.

*To learn more about *Beauty&Body Protein*, as well as my other Dr. Phoenyx brand nutritional supplements for healthy hair growth and fit body, go to DRPHOENYX.COM.

4. FOLLOW A REGULAR HAIR REGIMEN

Whether it's once a week or three times a week, you need to set a healthy regimen that involves regularly cleansing and conditioning your hair and scalp. The frequency and type of routine will differ from person to person. Some people may feel the need to frequently cleanse and condition their hair. Some people may not. Every person and head of hair is different, and truthfully there's no universal routine that you need to stringently follow. The routine should be set in accordance to your lifestyle. The overall point of cleansing and conditioning is to allow your hair to grow in a relatively clean and healthy environment. This is done by maintaining a schedule where you are keeping your hair and scalp free from excessive dirt, oil and product buildup.

5. INCORPORATE REGULAR SCALP MASSAGES

Stress is a major cause of imbalance and even hair loss. This is why scalp massages are an important part of growing hair. Scalp massages will help to relieve stress and trigger the release of feel-good hormones like dopamine and serotonin. Scalp massages will also stimulate blood flow to hair follicles, which is vital for hair growth. Scalp massages can be easily done on a daily basis. I give myself a daily scalp massage for at least two to three minutes at a time. When massaging my scalp, I like to use carrier oils like peppermint that soothe and stimulate blood flow. Also, scalp massages don't have to be a solo activity. For the married or coupled-up folks, this is a great time to get a little closer to the one you love. Scalp massages can be used as a wonderful time to create intimacy while putting your loved one's hands to great use!

6. EXERCISE

Remember, healthy hair comes from a healthy body. Exercise stimulates hair growth, and has the added benefit of reducing stress. So, whether it's walking, jogging, swimming or yoga, make sure to make time for exercise. Exercise is an important component to health and hair.

7. BE MINDFUL OF COMBS & BRUSHES

Many of us grew up following hair care practices that were actually doing more harm than good. One of those practices is brushing. Women usually brush their hair because they've been told these three things about brushing:

- Brushing your hair will stimulate scalp circulation and thus, stimulate hair growth

- Brushing your hair will help distribute natural oils (i.e. sebum) to the ends of your hair

- Brushing is necessary for proper grooming and preventing tangles

I grew up hearing all of these things about brushing. I also heard the myth that brushing hair one hundred times a day was the best way to grow healthy hair. While I did regularly brush my hair, I must admit that I never did believe that whole 'one hundred times a day' thing. I just never thought it made much sense. I mean really, what's the difference between brushing twenty times versus one hundred times- other than a pretty sore scalp?

The thing about brushes is that they end up doing more harm than good on afro-textured hair. Yes, the rounded bristles on some brushes can massage and simulate the scalp, but you don't need a brush to stimulate blood flow to the scalp. You can get the same affect by simply using your fingers to gently massage your scalp. Secondly, brushes don't effectively distribute sebum to the ends of hair. Afro-textured hair, because of its coils and bends, will naturally inhibit the flow of sebum to the ends of the hair, period. Brushing will not counteract this. If you want the ends of your hair to get the benefits of oil, all you have to do is smooth oil on the ends of your hair. Jojoba oil is excellent hair oil because it has a very similar molecular and chemical composition to sebum. Personally, I think smoothing a little jojoba oil on the ends of my hair is a much better alternative to literally ripping my hair shaft apart with a brush.

Finally, brushing does not prevent tangles. The truth is actually quite the opposite. The act of brushing produces a sheering effect against the cuticle, resulting in damage and hair that will become more prone to tangling as time goes on. When your cuticles are damaged from brushing, or anything for that matter, the raised and jagged cuticles will snag on each other like Velcro. This promotes tangling. So brushing, because it damages and raises the cuticle, can actually make tangling worse in the long run.

All of the above are reasons why I have retired my hairbrush. You can brush your hair if you want, but you don't need it to stimulate your scalp. You don't need it to keep your hair oiled. And you certainly don't need it to detangle your hair. If you're still not convinced and absolutely feel like you need a brush to manage your hair I would advise you to check out the Denman brush. There are many women with afro-textured hair that report positive results with this brand of hairbrush. However, I have never used the Denman so I can't personally attest to its quality. I do *occasionally* use a plastic wide-toothed comb and I would recommend this type of hair tool to any woman with afro-textured hair who absolutely desires a comb.

Needless to say I do think women can rely too heavily on hair tools and increase the rate of damage to their hair as a result. If you are one of these women, I'd encourage you to back off from combs/brushes a bit and start using your hands more. Trust me, there's a lot of magic working in your fingers. Most of the time, I solely use my hands when cleansing, conditioning and styling my hair. Overall I've found that I can be a lot gentler with my hair when doing so.

8. ALWAYS SLEEP WITH A SATIN/SILK HAIR COVERING

You should always protect your hair at night by wearing a satin or silk bonnet to bed. You need to do this because cotton or nylon pillowcases are very absorbent and have the ability to literally suck moisture from your hair. Then, there's the issue of hair tangling when you sleep with your hair loose and uncovered. A major key to growing longer hair is protection. You want to protect your hair more than you are damaging it. Simply rubbing your hair against pillowcases and sheets can result in cuticle damage. Satin and silk head covers prevent this. Using a head cover will protect your cuticles from damage and it will also help your hair retain moisture. I know many women who have noticed a complete turn-around in the condition of their hair when they started covering it at night. Always remember to sleep with a satin or silk bonnet. Your hair will love you for this in the morning!

9. BE MORE MINDFUL OF PRODUCT USE

We have already determined that certain commercial hair product ingredients can damage your hair. This is why I suggest reading labels and learning as much about product ingredients as possible. There are many wonderful commercial products to choose from and it's ultimately up to you to choose your products wisely. I will offer a few basic tips on how to better choose your commercial hair products in a later chapter.

10. MINIMIZE OR COMPLETELY ELIMINATE HEAT STYLING

I put away flatirons, curling irons, and blow dryers years ago and haven't touched them since. After I did that, I noticed a complete turnaround in my hair. Besides chemicals, I also learned that heat styling is significantly damaging to hair. I used to be a chronic heat styling offender. Once I decided that I would start loving my hair, I decided to turn my back on a lot of previous hair practices. I figure that if growing hair is about love, then chronic heat styling is hate. I've learned that heat styling is completely counterproductive to my hair's growth and health. The only time you may catch me using heat is when I occasionally apply mild heat to my hair during deep conditioning treatments. Other than that, I don't use heat.

For some women with afro-textured hair, totally giving up heat is not an option. In those cases I'll offer a few suggestions to help minimize the damage your hair will incur from heat styling. Here are my suggestions:

KEEP HEAT STYLING TO A MINIMUM

Heat will leech moisture from your hair and dry your hair out. Dry hair will lead to breakage. Breakage will ultimately lead to hair that doesn't appear to grow. Remember, in order to grow hair longer, you must damage your hair at a slower rate than it is growing. If longer hair is your goal, you will need to keep heat styling to a minimum and preferably no more than once a week.

ONLY USE HEAT ON CLEAN HAIR

Heat from appliances can literally melt dirt and product buildup onto the cuticle. Thus, you should not use heat appliances on hair that's dirty, sweaty, or hair that has not been recently cleansed. Also make sure to regularly cleanse the surface of your heat appliances. The heating surfaces of appliances will get dirty over time, so keep them clean before using on hair.

KEEP THE HEAT LEVEL TO A MINIMUM

Unfortunately, settings on heat appliances are very arbitrary and there's no guarantee that a low setting is significantly safer than a medium or high setting. Furthermore, operating temperatures can range across different appliances. For example, one appliance on a low setting may have a temperature of 100°F (38°C), while the same low setting on another appliance may have a temperature of 125°F (52°C). This can create somewhat of a tricky hair situation. Thus, the most tactful approach is to use your appliance on the lowest possible setting while paying very close attention to how your hair reacts to the heat. Most importantly, use common sense.

If you notice smoke or a burning smell when you're using your appliance, then the heat is too high.

USE HEAT PROTECTANTS

You should never use heat on dry or naked hair. Before using a heat appliance, hair should be first coated with a heat or thermal protectant. This thermal protectant will serve as a buffer between your hair and direct heat. Heat protectants can range from commercial products with synthetic ingredients to more natural products like grapeseed oil.

USE A DIFFUSER WITH YOUR BLOW DRYER

When blow-drying hair, some women tend to start with hair that is too wet and/or concentrate heat on one section of the hair until it's bone dry before moving along to the next. This is not good. Blow-dryers use a combination of heat and high velocity air, which are both very drying and damaging to the cuticle and the hair shaft. In order to cut back on the length of time that hair needs to be exposed to heat to dry, it is wise to blot as much excess water from hair *before* blow-drying. Furthermore, when using a blow-dryer, it's best to stay on the lowest heat setting, evenly distribute the warm air rather than concentrate heat on just one area of the hair at a time, and most importantly, do not over-dry hair. In addition to these tips, it's best to use a diffuser with your blow-dryer. Diffusers are large, funnel shaped attachments that have the ability to evenly distribute heated air over a larger surface area. Using a diffuser does not mean your hair will be totally protected from heat damage. But, using a diffuser properly will help to reduce the damaging effects of blow-dryers.

A WORD ON CHEMICAL PROCESSING

Chemical processing weakens hair by breaking its protein bonds. Furthermore, using multiple chemical processes such as chemical straighteners and permanent dyes will have a significant damaging effect

CHAPTER 6
NUTRITION AND HAIR GROWTH

I am constantly emphasizing the intricate relationship between health and hair because I want you to fully understand and appreciate that you cannot be unhealthy and expect to have longer and fuller hair. It's just not going to happen. If you do things to improve your overall health, it will be reflected in your hair, as well as your outward appearance. In fact, proper nutrition as well as exercise are two very important (and often neglected) factors in healthy hair growth. If you exercise and eat right, you will grow healthier and stronger hair – *100% guaranteed!* Bottom line, healthy hair starts from the inside – from the foods you eat. And no shampoo or conditioner can ever fully substitute for a healthy diet. Unfortunately many women don't fully appreciate the crucial role nutrition and healthy living play in hair growth – *and beauty in general for that matter!*

That's why I decided to dedicate an entire chapter of my book to the topic of Nutrition. Truth be told, as a Sports Medicine Specialist I *absolutely* love talking nutrition, and through my medical and professional training, I have obtained a deep understanding and great appreciation for the role that foods and supplements play in both beauty and fitness. And of course, I want to share this knowledge with you as well, so that you can also achieve all your hair goals! So now I'm going to break down, in simple terms, why what we eat is so important in regards to hair growth, why protein is the most important nutrient in regards to hair growth, what other vitamins, minerals, and nutrients you should get in your diet for healthy hair, and I'll also touch on how nutritional supplements can also help you achieve your heathy hair goals.

MACRONUTRIENTS & MICRONUTRIENTS

The reason why our hair is so greatly affected by what we eat, and is ultimately a reflection of what we eat is because hair is primarily formed from the nutritional building blocks obtained from food. And in the most basic sense, the nutrients in our food can be broken down into two major categories: macronutrients and micronutrients. "Macro" means big and "micro" means small – so another way of thinking about macronutrients and micronutrients is simply "big nutrients" versus "small nutrients." There are countless types of micronutrients such as vitamins, minerals and antioxidants. Overall, these are all types of small-sized nutrients or *micronutrients* – whereas the bigger sized nutrients or *macronutrients* that make up the bulk of our food will be of three types: fat, carbohydrates, and protein.

Suffice to say, the topic of nutrition can get somewhat complicated and because I want to keep this information as *simple and as helpful as possible* what I'm going to do is give you my very special *Dr. Phoenyx Crash Course in Nutrition*, which will easily breakdown the most important takehome points I want you to have when it comes to how you can use nutrition to achieve healthy hair growth. So now let's talk fat, carbs, and the most important beauty nutrient – protein!

Frequently misunderstood, the macronutrient *fat* gets a lot of flak because the mere word itself – *fat* – tends to make people think they're eating something that probably isn't very good for them. But that's far from the case, because truth be told, fat is a wonderful nutrient that helps keep us healthy and our hair beautiful! Basically, there are *good fats* and *bad fats*, and for simplicity's sake, *good fats* are good for us because they help our bodies in countless ways. For example, fat is used to make sebum, which is a natural lubricant produced by our scalp that helps protect hair and give it a lovely shine. In fact, not getting enough fat in your diet and a deficiency in essential fatty acids, like omega-3 fatty acids can result in decreased sebum production, dry scalp, dry hair, and even hair loss. And not to stray too far from the topic of hair, but you might be surprised to learn that there are even some types of fat in foods that can help us burn belly fat! So bottom line, when it comes to fat, you shouldn't fear eating it at all, and you should do your best to make sure your diet includes a healthy dose of fat from whole food sources such as meat, dairy, nuts, and healthy oils like coconut oil.

Our next macronutrient are carbohydrates and they are mainly found in whole grains, vegetables, and fruits. Carbohydrates are a type of "fast fuel source" because they are most rapidly broken down into simple sugar, or glucose, which our body then uses for energy. When it comes to hair, carbohydrates don't really play a major role. But it's still important to keep in mind that a diet high in sugar and refined carbohydrates, like candies and other sweets, can negatively affect your hair due to the fact that sugar can cause hormonal and metabolic problems that can stunt hair growth and even cause your hair to fall out. So the simple takehome when it comes to carbs is to avoid unhealthy sources of carbs like sweets and highly processed foods, and maintain a diet that is rich in healthy carbs sources like vegetables, fruit, beans, nuts, and whole grains. This will help keep your body healthy overall, which means your hair will grow healthy too.

PROTEIN

Last but not least, we've come to our final and most important macronutrient when it comes to hair growth – protein! And actually, that statement alone doesn't quite give protein all the credit it deserves, because when it comes down to it, **protein is the foundation of beauty, health and fitness**. Really there is no other nutrient that comes close.

And here's the simple reason why: *Because protein is the primary building block of our hair, skin, nails.*

93

As I stated before, our hair is over 90% protein. Or skin, which is our body's largest and most important organs, is primarily made of protein. In addition to that, proteins are used to build many of your body's other organs. Protein is also used to make hormones, which are directly responsible for influencing hair growth and the hair growth cycle. Even our muscles are primarily made of protein!

Suffice to say, protein is literally everywhere in our body, and this is why protein plays the starring role in *beauty* and *health*. In fact, if your diet is deficient in protein, that deficiency *alone* can negatively affect your hair growth, and here are a few tell-tale signs that you aren't getting enough protein in your diet:

- Slow-growing hair, thinning hair, and hair that breaks easily
- Brittle and slow-growing nails
- Premature wrinkles, dull and dry-looking skin
- Poor and "flabby" muscle tone with weight loss
- Constant cravings for sweets and unhealthy foods
- Weakness and fatigue, especially during exercise

Now on the most basic level, protein is made up of small building blocks called *amino acids,* which are linked together in a chain-like configuration to form a full protein. Altogether, there are 20 different types of amino acids, nine of which are considered essential because our bodies cannot produce them on its own, and therefore these *essential amino acids* must be obtained through our diet. Foods like meat, eggs, dairy, quinoa, and my nutritional supplement *Beauty&Body Protein,* are all highly desirable because they contain *complete proteins,* which is just another way of saying that the proteins in these types of foods will contain all 20 amino acids. Keep in mind too that not all proteins are created equal. For example, many plant food sources will not contain all 20 amino acids and will instead contain *incomplete proteins,* which means that if you're vegetarian it's very important that you mix and match your food sources to ensure that you do get enough complete proteins in your diet.

Bottom line, your hair and your body need protein – lots of it! So whether you eat meat or are strictly vegetarian, make sure you maintain a diet that contains lots of protein-rich food sources like chicken, fish, seafood, lamb, beef, eggs, legumes (beans), tofu, grains, nuts, seeds, and dairy.

VITAMINS, MINERALS & ANTIOXIDANTS

Vitamins, minerals and antioxidants are known as micronutrients. These micronutrients can be found in food and are also essential for growing hair. Within the human body there are 13 vitamins that you need to maintain overall growth and function. Theses vitamins are sub classified as either *water-soluble* or *fat-soluble* vitamins. The 4 fat-soluble vitamins are vitamins A, D, E, and K. The 9 water-soluble vitamins are vitamin C and the eight B vitamins.

Minerals are also important micronutrients. There are numerous minerals that your body needs for growth and function. Calcium is one example of a mineral that is needed for hair growth. Micronutrients also include antioxidants. Antioxidants are substances that help protect the cells in your body from free radical damage. Free radicals are toxic and highly reactive molecules that are naturally produced by cells during periods of metabolism, breakdown and stress. Free radicals are damaging to other cells and are directly responsible for the aging process, as well as many other adverse health conditions. Antioxidants are basically micronutrients that help to stabilize cells and reverse the negative effects of free radical damage. They are also very helpful micronutrients and can come in many different forms with multiple functions. Some vitamins and minerals also function dually as antioxidants. For example selenium, as well as vitamins A, C, E and B6, are also well-known antioxidants.

Together micronutrients and macronutrients all help to stimulate hair growth, prevent hair loss, maintain the health of our scalp, and protect our hair from damage. It's also important to know that micronutrients and macronutrients rarely work independently of each other. For example, it is estimated that 10% of American women are iron-deficient. An iron deficiency can lead to iron deficiency anemia- a very common cause of hair loss in women. In order to prevent iron deficiency anemia, and prevent hair loss, you would also need to have a diet that is rich in vitamin B2. This is because Vitamin B2 is necessary for iron absorption. Without vitamin B2, your body would have a hard time absorbing iron from food. Thus, to prevent iron deficiency, and maintain healthy hair growth, you need a diet that is balanced in other nutrients besides just iron.

WATER

Water is another important nutrient, accounting for approximately 60% to 70% of the body's weight. Overall, our body needs a healthy, daily dose of water in order to function optimally and water intake is tied to hair growth.

Each day your body is losing water through sweat, urine, and other metabolic function. The average person can lose about 10 cups of water per day through sweat and urination alone!

In order to maintain internal fluid balance, you must replace the water your body loses. If you don't, you will become dehydrated. Dehydration is not only bad for your hair, it's also bad for your body, particularly your kidneys. Furthermore, dehydration is a state that doesn't necessarily have to be accompanied with extreme thirst, and many people can be significantly dehydrated, while not even realizing it.

To prevent dehydration and maintain healthy functioning, we're often told to drink several glasses of water per day to stay healthy and hydrated. But how much water is really enough?

Adequate water intake can be accomplished by drinking certain liquids and by eating certain foods that naturally contain water, such as fresh vegetables. As for fresh water intake, interestingly enough, many people follow or have heard of the "8-10 glass of water a day" rule. But, where did this rule come from and is it something you should follow? Actually, most doctors and nutritionists don't even know where that rule came from! It turns out that there's no medical basis for the "8-10 glasses of water a day" rule.

The more appropriate rule is to just drink fresh water regularly and make sure you stay properly hydrated throughout the day. It's not as stringent as 8-10 glasses of water a day, and water intake requirements do vary from person to person. If you're not sure about your overall state of hydration, one of the easiest ways to tell if you're properly hydrated is by looking at your urine. If your urine is a pale yellow to clear, you're most likely hydrated. If your urine is a dark yellow, then you need to increase your water intake.

NUTRITIONAL SUPPLEMENTS- WHY THEY WORK

In a perfect world we would live the healthiest lifestyles and we would only eat the most nutritious foods. Thing is, we don't live in a perfect world and we're not perfect beings. Furthermore, nowadays many of us are functioning under very hectic schedules and lead lifestyles that make it more difficult to eat healthy all the time. From skipping meals to grabbing unhealthy, fast foods because they're more convenient, life sometimes gets in the way of living healthy and thus we end up eating foods that lack many key nutrients. In addition to that, many of our "healthy foods" don't pack as much of a nutritional punch due to the fact that many of today's foods are largely mass produced, sprayed with unhealthy chemicals like pesticides, and even the soil that we grow our food in contains less nutrients than it did 50 years ago.

Fortunately, this is where nutritional supplements like hair vitamins come into play, and can be a literal lifesaver for your hair growth. And for anyone looking to maintain grow health hair – if you haven't done so already – I think that's a very smart idea to start incorporating nutritional supplements into your diet and haircare regimen. To learn more about and order my advanced nutritional supplements for healthy hair growth, *Beauty&Body Protein* and *Natural Beauty*, go to DRPHOENYX.COM. And if you'd like to learn even more about how to eat to achieve your beauty goals – from healthy, gorgeous hair to flawless, supple skin, also check out my e-book guide, FitBeauty 101: Eat Your Way to Healthy Hair & Body.

Now as promised earlier in the book, here's a lil' treat that I wanted to share for all the foodies. Below is one of my favorite *Beauty&Body Protein* green smoothie recipes that I drink daily, usually for breakfast and/or after my workouts. It tastes incredibly yummy, is packed with healthy hair and body nutrients, and it's superfast and super easy to make. *Enjoy!*

DR. PHOENYX'S B&B GREEN SMOOTHIE

Ingredients

1 serving of Beauty&Body Protein (1 scoop)

2 cups of raw spinach

½ medium sized green apple

2 cups unsweetened coconut milk (can substitute with 3/4 cup plain Greek yogurt + 1/4 cup water)

Preparation: Mix all ingredients in blender to smooth consistency. Drink and enjoy!

Last but not least, let's close things out with a comprehensive list of specific vitamins and minerals that contribute directly to healthy hair growth, as well as the foods that naturally contain them. You can find these healthy hair growth vitamins, minerals and foods on the following two tables.

Table 1 - Vitamins for Healthy Hair Growth

Vitamin	Food Sources	Hair Benefits	Upper Tolerable Limit (UL)
Vitamin A (Retinol) *is an antioxidant	eggs, dried apricots, guava, pink grapefruit, cantaloupe, sweet potato, carrots, pumpkin, seafood, spinach, kale, dark green/yellow/red vegetables, fortified cereals	Regulates sebum production	3,000 mcg/day or 10,000 IU/day
Vitamin B-1 (Thiamin)	asparagus, romaine lettuce, mushrooms, spinach, sunflower seeds, tuna, green peas, tomatoes, eggplant, fortified rice, bread, cereals, and oats	Essential for growth of hair and skin	Unknown
Vitamin B-2 (Riboflavin)	dairy products, avocados, mushrooms, spinach, sun-dried tomatoes, sesame seeds, almonds, liver, fish, bread & wheat products, fortified cereals	Prevents dandruff. Helps prevent iron deficiency (anemia), a common cause of hair loss	Unknown
Vitamin B-3 (Niacin)	lean meats, liver, poultry, fish, tuna, bacon, cheese, nuts, peanuts, prunes, potatoes, sun-dried tomatoes, asparagus, fortified cereals	Stimulates blood flow to the hair follicle	35 mg/day *There is no upper limit for niacin intake when obtained via natural food sources*
Vitamin B-5 (Pantothenic Acid)	beef, chicken, liver, eggs, salmon, clams, royal jelly, rice, avocados, grains, nuts, dates, dried figs, prunes, watermelon, apricots, banana	Stimulates hair growth and prevents hair loss	Unknown
Vitamin B-6 (Pyridoxine) *is an antioxidant	cocoa powder, legumes, fish, cheese, whole grains, bread, pizza, green leafy vegetables, cauliflower, egg, cheese, banana, avocado, dates, figs, prunes, nuts	Stimulates hair growth and prevents hair loss	100mg/day

Biotin (Vitamin B-7)	almonds, cashews, peanuts, peanut butter, mushrooms, avocado, brown rice, lentils, bulgur, oats, beef, liver, nuts, egg yolks, chicken, soybeans, sardines, milk, mayonnaise	Helps to produce keratin and strengthen the hair shaft. May prevent hair loss and premature graying	Unknown
Folic Acid (Vitamin B-9)	avocado, apricots, dates, orange, pineapple, liver, grains, nuts, yeast, dark/green leafy vegetables, brown rice, almonds, peanuts, peanut butter, soybeans (edamame), sunflower seeds	Promotes cell renewal for hair and skin growth	1,000 mcg/day *There is no upper limit for folic acid intake when obtained via natural food sources*
Vitamin B-12 (Cobalamin)	cheese, beef, lamb, liver, egg yolks, crab, clams, seafood, sardines, salmon, oysters, herring, dried milk, mayonnaise	Stimulates hair growth	Unknown
Choline Bartrate (part of B vitamins)	soybeans, egg yolk, butter, peanuts, potatoes, cauliflower, lentils, oats, sesame seeds, flax seeds	Keeps the hair root moist	3,500 mg/day
Vitamin C (Ascorbic acid) *is an antioxidant	oranges, pineapples, strawberries, raspberries, blueberries, blackberries, spinach, kale, green leafy vegetables, tomatoes, red pepper, green bell peppers, cauliflower, marmalade, jam	Assists in the formation of a protein, a key component in the formation skin and hair	2,000 mg/day
Vitamin E (alpha-tocopherol) *is an antioxidant	egg, almonds, pistachio nuts, avocado, mango, blackberries, tuna, potato, sweet potato, spinach, peanut butter, mayonnaise, salad dressing	Encourages hair growth by enhancing blood circulation to the scalp	1,500 IU/day or 1,000 mg/day *There is no upper limit for vitamin E intake when obtained from natural food sources*

* Abbreviations: IU= international units; mg=milligrams; mcg=micrograms (1 µg=1mg).

* Unknown means a UL has not been established by the IOM.

* Many of the B vitamins influence healthy hair growth. There are a total of 8 B vitamins and they are referred to collectively as B complex vitamins. When you see a supplement that reads "B Complex" on the label, it simply means that it contains all 8 B vitamins.

Table 2 - Minerals for Healthy Hair Growth

Mineral	Food Sources	Hair Benefits	Upper Tolerable Limit (UL)
Calcium	apricots, almonds, berries, lemons, figs, milk, cheese, yogurt, tofu, oatmeal, seafood, spinach, kale, okra, cabbage, collards, broccoli, soy beans	Strengthens the hair shaft	2,500 mg/day
Copper	liver, shellfish, nuts, dry beans, oats, raisins, cocoa powder, peanut butter, broccoli, mushrooms, spinach, garlic, avocados, apricot, banana, peach	Helps hair maintain its natural color	10,000 mcg/day
Iodine	iodized salt, seafood, garlic, meat, milk, egg, cheese	Regulates thyroid hormone, which also affects hair growth	1,100 mcg/day
Iron	raisins, figs, avocado, liver, meats, eggs, nuts, grains, raisins, cocoa powder, green leafy vegetables, beets, beans, soybeans, seafood, fortified cereals	Helps prevent hair loss due to iron deficiency	45 mg/day
Manganese	liver, green vegetables, beans, grains, egg yolks, nuts, seaweed, pineapple	Stimulates growth of the hair and nails	11 mg/day
Selenium *is an antioxidant	seafood, meat, broccoli, onions, tomatoes, yeast, corn oil, brown rice, molasses	Strengthens the hair shaft	400 mcg/day
Silicon (Silica)	leafy green vegetables, asparagus, lettuce, cabbage, onions, sunflower seeds, cucumbers, oats, rice, whole grains, citrus fruits	Helps strengthen the hair shaft. A deficiency in silica is linked to brittle nails and hair	Unknown. However long-term use or very high doses has been linked to irreversible kidney damage
Zinc	shellfish, liver, poultry, nuts, egg yolks, cheese, lamb, beef, peanuts, walnuts, almonds, peanut butter soy beans, beans, lentils, peas	Stimulates hair growth and maintains hair's natural color	40 mg/day

* Abbreviations: mg=milligrams; mcg=micrograms (1 mcg= 1 µg).

* Unknown means a UL has not been established by the IOM.

TAKE HOME POINTS

For healthy hair growth, maintain a healthy, protein-rich diet that contains lots of protein-rich food sources like chicken, fish, seafood, lamb, beef, eggs, legumes (beans), tofu, grains, nuts, seeds, and dairy.

Take high quality nutritional supplements to ensure a healthy diet and to maximize hair growth potential. Order Dr. Phoenyx's advanced nutritional supplements for healthy hair growth at DRPHOENYX.COM.

Be sure to regularly drink water, especially when taking vitamins and other nutritional supplements.

If you are pregnant or have a medical condition, consult with your physician first before using a nutritional supplement.

CHAPTER 7
CATEGORIZING HAIR PRODUCTS

Hair products can be broken down into two broad categories: natural and commercial products. Natural products are those that come straight from the earth and are minimally processed before distribution. Natural products come from plants and animals. Unlike natural products, commercial products are synthetic and more refined. The average shampoo is an example of a commercial product. A few examples of natural products are extra virgin olive oil, unrefined shea butter, pure essential oils, and emu oil (emu oil is actually made from the fat of the emu, a bird native to Australia).

Natural products are excellent for improving hair's health and its growth potential. More specifically, plant-based natural products are beneficial because they feed hair nutrients to help with moisture retention and fortification. They also supply nutrients that have the ability to protect hair from harmful agents like UV-A and UV-B rays.

Time and time again, Mother Nature has proved to know what is best for our bodies, and our hair. Many plant-based products are rich in antioxidants, phytonutrients, phytochemicals and photo-protective compounds. These types of nutrients have been shown to be vital for sustaining human life, protecting the body, and preventing disease. I regularly use natural and plant-based products for their health benefits, and for the simplicity of it all. With natural products I like that I don't have to worry about reading through tons of ingredients in the product label. I can just pick up some unrefined shea butter and always know that my product will contain one ingredient- shea butter. Another added benefit of using natural products is that it allows for multi-tasking. Meaning, I can typically use natural products on other parts of my body besides my hair. For instance, most of the natural oils that I use on my hair can be easily used to condition my skin.

I do use a few commercial products for my hair care, but believe me when I tell you I do my research first. When possible, I also like to infuse my commercial products with natural ingredients like essential oils and Ayurvedic products.

Despite commercial product use, I must admit that I tend to rely more heavily on natural products. I like that natural products are simple and have many uses, but I also rely on them because there are commercial hair care products that contain ingredients that can be harmful to our hair, scalp and even our health. I'm not going to tell you that you should avoid commercial products altogether because I don't do that myself. However, I would encourage you to use as many natural products as you can. Furthermore, if you use commercial products, I would also advise you to pay attention to the product ingredients. Overall, you just want to use the products that are best for your health and your hair.

CLEANSERS & CONDITIONERS

Hair products can be broken down into two other basic categories: cleansers and conditioners. Cleansers are products that are designed to remove dirt, excess oil, and product buildup. Cleansers include commercial shampoos, some commercial conditioners, and natural soaps like castile soap (castile soap is derived from olive oil). While cleansers tend to be straightforward in what they do, the category of conditioners can be a bit more complex.

The term "hair conditioner" is inclusive of many types of hair products that alter the texture and appearance of hair. When I use the term *hair conditioner* I'm using a very generic term that includes many types of products. Thus, a *hair conditioner* and a *commercial conditioner* are not exactly the same thing. A commercial conditioner is your typical name brand conditioner that is used after a shampoo. On the other hand, hair conditioners are actually a very broad category of products, most of which are simply natural and commercial products that work to improve the condition of your hair by supplying it with things like moisture and protein.

Rarely will the average person ever need to use all of these types of hair conditioner products. I certainly haven't had to do this in order to achieve longer and healthier hair. Furthermore, I shy away from excessive product use because I've found that it increases the risk of product buildup, hair damage, and exposure to too many agents and chemicals. I like to keep things simple for my life and my hair. So, when caring for my hair, I choose products from these five basic categories of hair conditioners.

MOISTURIZERS

What they are: Moisturizers improve the elasticity of hair. Examples of simple, natural moisturizers are pure water (the ultimate moisturizer) and aloe vera gel. Any product that gives your hair an appreciable amount of water is a moisturizer. Water is usually the principle ingredient in commercial moisturizing products.

How often you should use: Moisturizing is one of the most important steps in caring for your hair. In fact, it is so important that I'd advise you do this step every single day. In addition to daily moisturizing, you also want to regularly condition your hair with a moisturizing deep conditioning treatment. Our hair tends to be drier than other hair types. Afro-textured hair needs a constant supply of moisture in order to maintain its elasticity. When hair is more elastic it can be more easily manipulated without breaking. If you're trying to grow your hair longer, then you will need to maintain its moisture content and elasticity. You should never put your hair in a state where it is deprived of moisture. Dryness is the number one cause of breakage in afro-textured hair.

HUMECTANTS

What they are: Humectants are moisturizers that work by pulling water from one area to another. When used appropriately, humectants have the ability to pull moisture from the surrounding air into hair. A few simple, natural humectants are honey, panthenol (vitamin B5), and vegetable glycerin.

How often you should use: Humectants can be used daily, but daily use may not always be a wise choice. While humectants may seem very appealing for moisturizing hair, you need to remember that humectants work by pulling water from one area to another. Humectants can pull moisture into hair, but they can also pull moisture away from hair under certain weather conditions. For example, if the surrounding air is drier than your hair, humectants can actually draw moisture away from your hair. I like using humectants because of their wonderful moisturizing capabilities, but I'm also careful about when and how often I use them. In a later chapter, I will give a more detailed explanation on how to best use humectants.

RECONSTRUCTORS

What they are: Reconstructors are products that contain protein, the major structural component of hair. The protein in these types of commercial products is usually in the form of hydrolyzed protein, which is basically protein that has been broken down into its smaller amino acid components. Reconstructors are commonly called protein treatments, and they help strengthen hair by introducing new protein that can bind to the structure of damaged hair through polymer crosslinking. These products rebuild the hair, hence the name "reconstructor." It's important to note that almost every commercial conditioner also contains some degree of protein or amino acids (protein building blocks) and can thus be thought of as a reconstructor. Examples of natural reconstructors are henna, wheat protein, soy protein and egg.

How often you should use: Reconstructors are further broken down into light protein and heavy protein treatments. The difference between a light versus heavy protein reconstructor lies in the size, type and concentration of protein molecules in the product. These differences will impact how well the protein binds to hair. All reconstructors do eventually wear off from hair after repeated washes, regardless of protein treatment type. Light protein treatments, which include things like commercial conditioners, leave-in conditioners and even curl activating sprays, tend to have a shorter lasting effect on hair than heavy protein treatments. Heavy protein treatments, which require the use of heat to facilitate protein binding, tend to bind more efficiently to hair and thus, have a longer-lasting reconstructing effect.

You won't actually find a product that's precisely labeled as a "light" or "heavy" protein treatment. However, you can easily tell the difference between a light and heavy protein treatment by the effect it has on hair. Light protein treatments rarely have a hardening effect on hair, while heavy protein treatments do. In fact, the hardening effect of a heavy protein treatment can be so profound that hair could literally snap if not handled appropriately. This hardening effect is the result of the significant shift in protein-moisture balance. As a result, you should always follow-up every heavy protein treatment with a moisturizing deep conditioning treatment. This will help to restore the protein-moisture balance to hair.

While protein treatments sound great for hair, it's important to be mindful of frequency of use. Most light protein treatments can be used often on hair (even daily in some cases). Heavy protein reconstructors or heavy protein treatments should not be used often because adding these types of heavier proteins to hair can have a very drying effect as the protein-moisture balance shifts to the protein side. This is why heavy protein treatments are generally recommended once every few weeks. Women with afro-textured hair should be especially careful when using heavy protein treatments. Remember, in most cases afro-textured hair will need more moisture than protein.

EMOLLIENTS

What they are: Emollients come in natural and synthetic form. Natural emollients are derived from living things, whereas synthetic emollients (e.g. mineral oil and petrolatum) are a byproduct of the distillation of crude oil. Silicone is also a type of synthetic emollient. Some people like to refer to emollients as *"moisturizers,"* and will use these two terms interchangeably. This is because emollients have a way of making our hair and skin *feel* moisturized. But, emollients are not moisturizers. Moisture is obtained from water and water-based products. Water is the ultimate moisturizer and emollients don't actually moisturize, they simply seal in moisture that's already there. So when placed on the hair shaft, an emollient will form a waterproof barrier and lock moisture in. There are a few natural emollients that can actually penetrate the hair shaft and provide extra conditioning to the hair, but most emollients will simply sit on the hair shaft. We'll get into those special conditioning emollients later. For right now, remember that emollients simply work by sealing in moisture. Examples of natural emollients are shea butter, olive oil and jojoba oil.

How often you should use: Emollients should always be used after moisturizing your hair. So if you moisturize daily, emollients should also be used on a daily basis. Not using an emollient after moisturizing will leave your hair more susceptible to moisture loss through evaporation. This is especially the case if you have highly porous hair. With that in mind, you should also never use an emollient on dry hair. Emollients seal moisture into hair, but they also block moisture out. Only use an emollient after you've moisturized your hair.

ACIDIFIERS

What they are: Acidifiers are also known as pH balancers. They are acidity regulators that help to restore the acid mantle. Your hair and skin's acid mantle can be altered by hair products, and acidifiers work to restore normalcy to the acid mantle. An acidifier will do two things: 1) restore pH balance to the acid mantle and 2) smooth out your hair cuticles. When the hair's acid mantle is maintained, the cuticle layer will remain flat and the protein bonds in the hair shaft will remain intact. Flat cuticles help to protect your hair, and they will also reflect light and give your hair sheen. Simple, natural acidifiers are an apple cider vinegar rinse or a lemon juice rinse.

How often you should use: Most commercial products already come slightly acidified, so pH balancing is not typically an issue. Still, many women like to make their own homemade acid rinses. These rinses work well for restoring the acid mantle, removing product buildup, smoothing the cuticle, and will often give hair more sheen, curl definition and bounce. Whenever you use a homemade acidifier rinse, you want to first dilute it with distilled water, and then use this as a final hair rinse after your hair has been thoroughly cleansed and conditioned. You don't have to wash out the acidifier rinse afterwards. The key thing to remember about homemade acid rinses is that you should only use a rinse of *diluted* acid. Never use pure, undiluted apple cider vinegar or lemon juice on hair. These liquids are very acidic and have the ability to breakdown the protein structure of your hair.

To make an acid rinse, I use one tablespoon of pure, organic apple cider vinegar for every cup of water. The frequency of acid rinse use is a personal choice, but I don't find it necessary to use this homemade acid rinse on my hair more than once a month. Ideally, you should also pH test your homemade products with pH testing strips before using on your hair.

A WORD ON HOMEMADE PRODUCTS

Personally, I've always enjoyed a more hands-on approach to my hair, and I do enjoy mixing homemade hair treatments. Maybe you're just like me and enjoy this too. But here's a bit of a warning. As fun as making hair products can be, it is still wise to exercise caution because there is the risk of contamination when making homemade products. Homemade products, unlike commercial products, tend to be made without preservatives that prevent the growth of fungi, mold, bacteria and other nasty microorganisms that can make you sick. Here are a few suggestions on how to safely make and use homemade products:

- Always use boiled or distilled water and a sterilized container for storing product.

- Make a small amount of homemade product to last for one week at a time.

- Date stamp and store all homemade products in the refrigerator when not in use.

- Consider adding the contents of a capsule of vitamin E to homemade products. Vitamin E acts as a preservative.

- Skin test for allergies before using any homemade products.

TAKE HOME POINTS

Hair products can be broken down into two broad categories: natural and commercial products. Natural products are those that come straight from the earth or animals. Commercial products contain synthetic or man-made ingredients.

Natural products are rich in antioxidants, phytonutrients, phytochemicals and photo-protective compounds that help to improve hair's health and its growth potential.

Hair products can be broken down into two other basic categories: cleansers and conditioners. Cleansers are products that are designed to remove dirt, excess oil, and product buildup. Cleansers include commercial shampoos, some commercial conditioners, and natural soaps like castile soap (castile soap is derived from olive oil). The term "hair conditioner" is inclusive of many types of hair products that improve the condition and appearance of hair.

Commercial conditioners are not the only type of hair conditioner. Hair conditioners include: moisturizers, humectants, reconstructors, emollients and acidifiers.

Exercise caution when making homemade hair products due to the risk of contamination by fungi, mold, bacteria and other microorganisms.

CHAPTER 8
NATURAL EMOLLIENTS

Natural emollients are fats derived from plants, nuts, seeds, fruits and even animals. When the fat takes on a solid form at room temperature, it will typically be referred to as butter. When the fat takes on a liquid form at room temperature, it will typically be referred to as oil. Interestingly enough, the terms "butter" and "oil" are not always very precise. For example, while coconut oil is actually solid at room temperature, it is still commonly referred to as an oil, and not butter.

Though I use a mix of natural and commercial products, I tend to rely exclusively on natural emollients. There is a specific reason for this. Natural butters and oils are rich in phytonutrients, antioxidants, vitamins, plant proteins and essential fatty acids, as well as other nutrients that will nourish hair and stimulate hair growth. In addition, natural emollients are less occlusive and less disruptive to the acid mantle of the hair and skin.

Along with all of these benefits, some natural emollients can also help to protect the hair shaft from protein loss. Protein loss occurs when the hair shaft loses protein due to damage, and this is precisely the reason for using a protein treatment. Giving your hair protein will reinforce its strength and structure. Besides protein treatments, there are also certain natural emollients that can penetrate the hair shaft, bind to the protein structure of the hair, prevent protein loss, and ultimately help to strengthen the hair.

Unfortunately, synthetic emollients, such as mineral oil, are often severely lacking in most of the nutrients and protective capabilities that I have outlined. Synthetic oils, like mineral oil, are excellent for sealing in moisture. However, they do tend to be very occlusive and can form a strong layer that blocks your skin's ability to eliminate toxins. They can also build up on hair and block moisture absorption. Furthermore, synthetic oils can only be washed from hair with stronger agents, such as sulfates. On top of all of that, some synthetic emollients may even have adverse health effects. This is why I favor natural emollients. You can use synthetic emollients to seal your hair if you want. It's all personal preference. From my own experience, I've consistently found that natural emollients are far superior in their ability to nourish my hair and skin.

PENETRATING & NON-PENETRATING EMOLLIENTS

There are a few natural emollients that can actually penetrate the hair, while others simply coat the surface of the hair and help to seal in moisture. Coconut oil is one example of an emollient that can penetrate hair. Many women have heard about the penetrating effect of certain emollients and make a conscious effort to only use these types of emollients. Often, these women assume that a penetrating emollient is simply "better." But does the ability to penetrate hair really make one emollient better than another?

While penetrating emollients do have their advantages, it certainly doesn't mean you should totally dismiss the advantages of non-penetrating emollients. Each type of emollient has its own benefits, thus making it better for different purposes. For example, penetrating emollients (like coconut oil) are especially useful *before* washing hair. It has been scientifically shown that penetrating oils will protect hair from becoming damaged by hygral fatigue and protein loss. This is because penetrating emollients are better absorbed into hair and prevent the hair from absorbing too much water. On the other hand, it has also been shown that non-penetrating emollients are better able to form a coat over hair that will effectively prevent water from evaporating out of the cortex. Thus, non-penetrating emollients are more useful *after* washing hair because they help to keep hair moisturized.

As you can see, it's not as easy as saying that one kind of emollient is generally better than another. Penetrating and non-penetrating oils do different things to benefit hair. Ultimately, you must first determine what your hair needs, then pick your emollient accordingly.

BUTTERS

Butters are primarily packaged as organic, unrefined or refined. When you see a butter that has been marked "organic," this is the most natural, raw form of butter. You can easily identify a raw butter because it is usually packaged generically and sold in a large, hard or mildly soft lump. This butter is pure. Nothing has been added to it and nothing has been removed. A certified organic butter will also carry a label by the United States Department of Agriculture (USDA) that ensures that it is 95-100% organic. If a butter (or product in general) does not carry this USDA seal, it has not been certified as organic.

Unrefined butter, on the other hand, has been processed, but the processing has been done without changing most of its nutrient and vitamin content. Lastly, refined butter has been more heavily processed through deodorization, bleaching, and other processes that strip away most of its nutritive properties.

When choosing butters, it's important to take note of whether it's organic, unrefined or refined. Then you should choose based on your personal preference. If you want something with most, if not all, of its nutrients, go with an organic or unrefined butter.

I have listed several natural emollients. These are just a few that have worked well for my hair. There are many more butters and natural emollients to choose from, so don't feel constrained by these lists. Furthermore, I don't want you to get too bogged down when choosing emollients either. Truth be told, many natural emollients have similar hair and skin benefits. So, just pick one or two and try them out. See how they work for you, and then commit based on how they work for your hair. You should also consider rotating your emollients based on the time of year or weather. That's what I do.

In addition, if you're someone who likes to heat your butters/oils for mixing purposes, be careful not to over-heat. Heating helps for whipping and mixing, but overheating can also diminish nutrient content. Most importantly, if you have allergies to plants or nuts, be careful about using certain natural emollients.

Cupuacu Butter is a rich, exotic butter with a soft, creamy consistency. It contains tons of nutrients, is a natural UV-A and UV-B ray protectant, and is excellent for sealing moisture into hair/skin.

Coffee Bean Butter is a rich emollient with a coffee-like aroma and a smooth, buttery consistency. It is rich in antioxidants, natural sunscreens, and is often used to treat dermatitis and inflammatory skin conditions.

Macadamia Nut Butter is a very light butter (and oil) that can be used to treat dry hair and damaged skin. Macadamia nut contains palmitoleic acid, a highly effective anti-aging compound.

Mango Butter is a light butter that is rich in vitamins A, C and E. These types of vitamins are all antioxidants that stimulate healthy hair growth while protecting the hair and scalp.

Murumuru Butter is a light butter that can penetrate the hair shaft and guard against hygral fatigue and protein loss.

Shea Butter is one of the heavier butters, and is often referred to as "Women's Gold" in Africa. African healers have been using shea butter for thousands of years to nourish hair and skin. Shea butter can be used "as is" but due to its heavy consistency, many women like to whip or mix shea butter before using on their hair.

Tucuma Butter is a light butter with a very pleasant caramel, coffee-like scent. This butter is very rich in vitamin A and easily penetrates skin on contact. Tucuma and murumuru butter belong to the same family of exotic Amazonian emollients.

CARRIER OILS & ESSENTIAL OILS

Just like butters, natural oils are also rich in antioxidants, vitamins, essential fatty acids and other nutrients that promote scalp health and healthy hair growth. Natural oils can be further broken down into carrier oils and essential oils.

Carrier oils, which are also known as *base oils* and *vegetable oils,* are often made from the fatty portion of a plant- usually the seeds, kernels or nuts. Carrier oils can also be made from animal fats. Essential oils are concentrated extracts taken from the aromatic parts of plants, usually the leaves, flowers or blossoms. Essential oils are easily distinguished from carrier oils by their more concentrated aroma and high volatility.

Carrier oils are excellent natural emollients and I use them often because they are versatile for mixing and easily distributed on hair. When purchasing carrier oil you want to always go for the best quality, which would be an organic oil. If you can't find an organic oil, get one that doesn't contain preservatives, artificial color, fragrance, parabens and synthetic oils. Also look for carrier oils that are unrefined and have been *cold pressed* or *cold processed.* These are the best quality oils. Cold pressed and cold processed means that the oil has been processed with minimal heat or no heat at all. Heating will alter oils, resulting in lower quality and efficacy. In addition to buying quality oils, make sure to only buy as much oil as you need at one given time. Also make sure to store carrier oils in a cool, dark place. Oils can go rancid, and exposure to air or sunlight will speed up the degradation process. One simple way to help extend the shelf life of oil is by mixing it with the contents of a single vitamin E capsule. Pure vitamin E is an antioxidant and natural preservative, which will help to keep the oil from going rancid as quickly. Still, most of the oils I listed below have a shelf life of one year or less and I would not keep them longer than that.

Aloe Vera Oil is a light, versatile oil (and gel). Aloe vera contains the enzyme superoxide dismutase, an antioxidant that has been shown in studies to prevent hair graying and stimulate hair growth.

Avocado Oil is a medium-to-heavy oil that can penetrate the hair shaft and protect hair from protein loss.

Camellia Oil is a light oil that comes from Japan and is also referred to as tea seed oil (not to be confused with tea tree oil). Camellia oil is very rich and works very well for reconditioning dry and/or damaged hair.

Castor Oil is a medium-to-heavy oil that can penetrate the hair shaft and is used to prevent thinning hair and promote healthy hair growth. Jamaican Black Castor oil is an unrefined and higher quality form of castor oil.

Coconut Oil is a medium-to-heavy oil that can penetrate the hair shaft, and protect hair from hygral fatigue and protein loss.

Olive Oil is a medium-to-heavy oil that can penetrate the hair shaft and is used for deep conditioning and preventing hair loss. Extra virgin olive oil is a higher quality, less refined form of olive oil.

Jojoba Oil is a very light, versatile and "hair friendly" oil that mixes very well with other products. Jojoba oil is also very similar to sebum in chemical and molecular composition.

Grapeseed Oil is a very light oil that can be easily mixed with heavier oils to help "lighten" their consistency for easier absorption by the hair and skin. Grapeseed oil also works well as a heat protectant.

Sweet Almond Oil is a light oil that mixes very well with other emollients and is quite inexpensive. Sweet almond oil is also used to help "lighten" the consistency of heavier oils.

Wheat Germ Oil is a light oil that also contains protein. Wheat germ oil can be used as a deep conditioning light protein treatment and as a heat protectant.

Which Oil Should You Use for Your Hair?

This is a very common question, especially with women who are new to using emollients. The answer mostly lies in personal preference. You should use whichever works for your hair. It's not an exact science and every head of hair is different. If you'd like a bit more direction, I would suggest these oils for sealing: aloe vera oil, camellia oil, grapeseed oil, jojoba oil, and sweet almond oil. For deep conditioning I would suggest these oils: avocado oil, camellia oil, castor oil, coconut oil, olive oil, and wheat germ oil.

ESSENTIAL OILS

Essential oils have been used for thousands of years to influence mood, induce healing and provide relaxation. Certain essential oils have also been used to stimulate blood flow, soothe the scalp and stimulate hair growth. Essential oils are very versatile (just like carrier oils) and can be easily added to other natural and commercial hair care products. Before using on skin, most essential oils need to first be diluted in carrier oil. In fact, carrier oils are named as such because they "carry" essential oils onto the skin. Essential oils are typically mixed with carrier oils for these two reasons: 1) pure essential oils are very potent and can actually irritate the skin when applied directly to it and 2) essential oils are very volatile, and can evaporate easily if not first stabilized in a carrier oil base.

Before using an essential oil, you should test a small area of your skin to make sure you are not sensitive or allergic. As a general guideline, you should just use a couple drops of essential oil at a time and dilute no more than 8-10 **total** drops of essential oil(s) in ½ cup of carrier oil. After diluting, place a few drops of the oil infusion on your fingertips and massage gently into your scalp. You can also warm your carrier oil and essential oil blend before massages. Many women like using warmed oils on their skin or scalp. To warm your oil, place the bottle or vial of oil into a bowl of warm water for a few minutes. Do not warm oils in the microwave or on stovetop. A gentle heating of the oil is all that is needed.

When not in use, essential oils should always be stored in dark glass bottles with tight fitting tops. Dark bottles are necessary because direct light can cause chemical changes to the oil. You should not store essential oils in plastic containers because they can dissolve the plastic and become contaminated. Finally, if you are pregnant or nursing, you should check with your physician before using essential oils.

Below are a few essential oils that promote scalp health and healthy hair growth. An asterisk next to an oil means that it is also commonly used to stimulate hair growth. You can find these essential oils, as well as the previous emollients, in major health food stores and via online distributors like Mountain Rose Herb and From Nature With Love.

Basil Oil*	Bay Leaf Oil*	Burdock Root Oil*
Clary Sage Oil*	Cedarwood Oil	Eucalyptus Oil
Grapefruit Oil*	Lavender Oil*	Lemon Oil
Lemongrass Oil	Patchouli Oil	Peppermint Oil*
Rose Oil	Rosemary Oil*	Sandalwood Oil
Tangerine Oil*	Tea Tree Oil*	Thyme Oil*
Ylang Ylang Oil		

TAKE HOME POINTS

Natural emollients, such as butters and oils, are fats derived from plants, nuts, seeds, fruits and animals. They are rich in phytonutrients, anti-oxidants, vitamins, plant proteins and essential fatty acids, as well as other nutrients that will nourish hair and stimulate hair growth. When compared to synthetic emollients (i.e. mineral oil), they tend to be more nutritive, less occlusive and less disruptive to the acid mantle of the hair and skin.

Synthetic oils, like mineral, are excellent for sealing in moisture. However, they do tend to be very occlusive and can build up on hair very easily. When cleansing hair of synthetic emollients, you will need to use stronger cleansing agents, such as shampoos containing sulfates.

Penetrating emollients (i.e. murumuru butter, avocado oil, castor oil, coconut oil) work well for protecting hair against hygral fatigue and protein loss. Non-penetrating emollients work well at sealing hair and keeping it moisturized.

When purchasing butters, look for those that are raw and organic. When purchasing carrier oils, look for those that are unrefined and have been cold pressed or cold processed.

Natural emollients, particularly oils, can go rancid. Exposure to air or sunlight will speed up the degradation process. One simple way to help extend the shelf life of natural oil is by mixing it with the contents of a single vitamin E capsule. Pure vitamin E is an antioxidant and natural preservative, which will help to keep the oil from going rancid as quickly.

Always dilute essential oils in carrier oil before directly applying to skin.

CHAPTER 9
HOW TO CHOOSE COMMERCIAL PRODUCTS

The key to choosing commercial products is to always read the ingredients on the label. Manufacturers will label all product ingredients in order, from the most abundant ingredient to the least abundant ingredient. When reading product ingredients, it's a good idea to follow the *Rule of Thirds*. The top third of the ingredients usually represents 90-95% of the product, the middle third usually represents 5-8% of the product, and the bottom third represents 1-3%. When selecting commercial shampoos, moisturizers and conditioners for your hair regimen, I'd also suggest that you specifically look for products that fit the criteria I've listed below.

SHAMPOO

It's best to use shampoos that are sulfate-free. Most product manufacturers will have something on their shampoo label that identifies them as "sulfate free." Sulfates, which are commonly used in commercial shampoos, are very harsh agents and extremely drying to hair. Sulfates commonly added to shampoos are sodium lauryl and laureth sulfates (SLS), ammonium lauryl and laureth sulfates (ALS), sodium myreth sulfate and TEA laureth sulfate. There are sulfate-free shampoos and then there are shampoos that are only free of individual sulfate types (i.e. "SLS-free" shampoos). An SLS-free shampoo could still contain a different type of sulfate, so be sure to check the ingredients label to verify if a shampoo is totally sulfate free.

CONDITIONER

When selecting commercial conditioners, you want to look for those that fit at least two of these three criteria:

1. Contains water as the most abundant ingredient.

2. Contains natural, plant-derived or botanical ingredients (e.g. aloe vera, coconut extract, fruit extract, etc.).

3. Is an organic product. A product that contains natural ingredients is not always organic. Certified organic products will always carry the USDA seal of approval.

It is actually very easy to find commercial conditioners and *even shampoos* that fit all three of these criteria. Furthermore, when possible it's always best to buy hair products that are organic because they gently infuse your hair follicles and skin cells with natural minerals, herbal extracts, and oils. One of the easiest ways to find these types of products is by shopping in stores like Whole Foods Market and Trader Joe's. While you can buy your commercial products from anywhere you like, I suggest these stores because they are known to hold high standards of quality that manufacturers must meet before a product can be sold in their stores.

If you'd like to learn more about the various ingredients in your hair and cosmetic products, as well as how to better pick commercial products, you should also check out these books, which are available at most public libraries:

Don't Go Shopping for Hair-Care Products Without Me by Paula Begoun

What's In Your Cosmetics: A Complete Consumer's Guide to Natural & Synthetic Ingredients by Aubrey Hampton

TAKE HOME POINTS

Use the Rule of Thirds to analyze product ingredients: The top third of the ingredients usually represents 90-95% of the product, the middle third usually represents 5-8% of the product, and the bottom third represents 1-3%.

Use sulfate-free shampoos.

Use conditioners that fulfill at least 2 out of these 3 criteria:

1. Contains water as the most abundant ingredient.

2. Contains natural, plant-derived or botanical ingredients.

3. Is an organic product (Certified organic products will always carry the USDA seal of approval).

CHAPTER 10
LABOR OF LOVE

I follow very simple, defined steps when cleansing, conditioning and styling my hair. I call this entire process my *labor of love*. I think the name is very fitting because it really does describe how I approach my hair in order to maintain growth, health and length. It takes work and lots of TLC to achieve longer and healthier hair. Love leads to growth.

Some women will find it difficult to achieve their hair goals because they don't fully understand the importance of being nurturing and protective. So, from this point on I'd like for you to think of your hair care regimen as a *labor of love*. This will remind you to put in an extra bit of work, patience and care into your hair in order to achieve the length you want.

My *labor of love* is very simple and broken down into seven steps: pre-cleansing, cleansing, deep conditioning, moisturizing, sealing, stimulating, and protective styling. You can follow this regimen exactly as I do, or you can tweak it a bit to fit your lifestyle. Overall, I think following most of these steps, as often as you can, will help you to achieve your hair goals.

PRE-CLEANSING

HOW OFTEN: BEFORE EVERY CLEANSE

Before I get to what pre-cleansing is, I wanted to make an announcement that from this point on, I'm going to refer to a pre-cleanse as a "pre-poo," and pre-cleansing as "pre-pooing." *I'll let you giggle like a little schoolgirl before I continue.*

Pre-pooing is the process of coating the hair with a "pretreatment" *before* actually cleansing the hair. The pretreatment is used to protect and nourish the hair shaft and prepare it for cleansing. Pre-pooing is done to give your hair extra conditioning, while also protecting it from the cleansing process itself. I know that sounds a bit weird, but yes, you do need extra conditioning and protection before you cleanse your hair. Why? The truth is that cleansing your hair comes with the risk of damage. Every time you cleanse your hair, you risk certain degrees of damage. This happens because hair is most fragile in its wet state. Overall, the extent of damage to wet hair can vary based on several factors, and pre-pooing can help to reduce the damage that hair incurs from the 3 H's: Hygral fatigue, Harsh cleansers, and a Helluva lot of tangles.

Hygral fatigue

As explained earlier, repeatedly wetting and drying the hair can cause damage via hygral fatigue. One way to control this type of damage is by doing a pre-poo. For instance, when you pre-poo with coconut oil (a penetrating emollient), the oil will penetrate the hair shaft and prevent water from oversaturating your hair. Water will enter the hair shaft, but not too much. Ultimately, you'll still get the cleansing and moisturizing effect from water, but you won't get the damaging effect from hygral fatigue.

Harsh Cleansers

You should avoid commercial cleansers with harsh agents like sulfates. Even sulfate-free shampoos, although more gentle, may still contain cleansers that have the ability to disturb the acid mantle and strip away natural oil from your hair. This is another reason why pre-pooing is effective. Pre-poo serves as a light buffer between your scalp, hair, and many harsh cleansing agents.

Helluva lot of tangles

Finally, pre-poo also helps to minimize tangles. It's inevitable that you'll get tangles when washing your hair because the process requires manipulation of the hair shaft. But, you can cut down on the amount of tangling by prepping your hair. And that's what pre-pooing is essentially. It's a hair prep. When you pre-poo, you will need to detangle your hair before applying product to it. You don't just want to apply pre-poo without detangling first because it is important to evenly coat all strands of your hair. Furthermore, initially detangling your hair will drastically minimize or even eliminate the amount of detangling you have to do once you've finished washing your hair.

HOW TO PRE-POO

Pre-pooing is broken down into three steps: sectioning hair, detangling and applying pre-poo. This process will take some time, especially if you have thicker, longer hair. In this case, you should not pre-poo when you're rushed. I like to pre-poo on nights when I can pour myself a glass of wine and watch *really good* bad reality TV. I do this because I know that performing this step while rushed, or even stressed, can result in not giving my hair the patience and finesse it needs. Remember, manipulating hair in itself will cause damage, but the amount of damage will be minimal if you're gentle and patient during the process.

STEP 1: SECTIONING HAIR

Before detangling, section your hair into four equal parts. I like to make two pigtails in the front and two pig tails in the back. I think working with four sections is very easy, but you can add more sections if you like. After sectioning hair, use a very soft scrunchie to tie off each section. Do not use rubber bands or elastic bands because they tend to snag on hair. You should also skip using a comb during this step. You don't need a comb to section or detangle your hair. All you need are your hands. Using your hands will drastically cut down on the damage done to your hair.

After you've loosely tied off each section, *lightly* mist your hair (especially the ends) with a spray that has detangling properties. Hair should NEVER be detangled dry. Dry hair is not as "elastic" and "stretchable" as wet hair. Dry hair is more likely to break under the tension of manipulation, and wetting hair gives it more flexibility for movement. In many cases, you can dually use your daily moisturizing spray as your detangling spray. The key characteristic of a good detangling spray is that it will give hair *slip*. Just spray your hair and gently rub the strands between your fingers to get the slip factor working. It is the slip factor that helps the hair shafts move easily past each other without much friction or snagging during the detangling process.

STEP 2: DETANGLING

After all of your hair has been moistened, untie one section at a time and begin detangling with your fingers. Work *gently* from the ends of your hair to the root. Once a section of hair is detangled, gently tie it off again with your scrunchie, and proceed to the next section of hair. Work on one section of hair at a time, and keep any section that you're not actively working on tied off.

How to Tangle With Tangles

During the detangling process, you may encounter a tangle here or there. It's inevitable so don't let tangles overly frustrate you. To deal with the inevitable tangle, you should follow these steps:

1. Lightly mist the tangle and wait a couple minutes.

2. Relax and have a few laughs watching *Real Basketball Housewives of Compton.*

3. After you've given you hair enough time to moisten, return to gently working on the tangle.

When detangling, gently try to slide as many strands of hair from the tangle as you can. Never pull or stretch your hair until the tangle pops- that's very damaging! No bueno!

If you've got a particularly stubborn tangle, it may help to use a fine sewing needle to help loosen knots. Just use the pointed end of the needle to navigate through the small loops of the knot. Gently use the needle and your fingers to work the tiny knots loose. This is a technique that I love to use for stubborn, small tangles. If you're skillful *and* gentle, you'll usually be able to get the entire tangle loose with a sewing needle.

In cases where skill *or* luck isn't on your side, you will need to trim the knot from your hair. Having to trim knots may be a bit annoying, but trust me, it's better to trim a knot immediately. You don't want to ignore it and risk more hair getting caught in it later.

To trim a knot, simply use a sharp pair of hair scissors. Your hair scissors should not be dull and they should not be used for anything other than your hair. When trimming hair, just make a clean, quick cut. Then rinse and dry your scissors. Make sure your scissors are clean after ever use and store them away.

Tangles and Knots- Are They Normal?
Occasional tangles and knots are normal. Fairy knots are another type of knot that can form on a single strand of hair (usually close to the ends). Fairy knots have a tendency to form on afro-textured hair that is frequently worn loose or not protectively styled.

Occasional tangles and knots aren't necessarily a sign of unhealthy hair, but frequent tangles and knots can be a nuisance and are a sign that the hair's cuticle is raised or possibly damaged. When cuticles are not flat or damaged, individual strands of hair will have a tendency to snag or catch on each other. This can lead to increased tangling and knotting.

STEP 3: APPLYING PRE-POO

Once all of your hair is detangled, start applying pre-poo to each section. This is best done by untying a section of hair, scooping up some pre-poo on your fingertips and applying it to your hair in a smoothing, downward motion from root to tip. Smoothing downward is done to evenly distribute pre-poo to your hair and it's also done to not disturb the natural orientation of your hair cuticles. Under normal conditions, cuticles are lying flat and in a downward direction. You may have to go against the orientation of your cuticle at times (i.e. when detangling), but for the most part you should try to manipulate your hair in a way that does not go against your cuticles. This is why smoothing your hair from root to tip is recommended.

If you have a lot of hair, applying a pre-poo treatment will take a few minutes. Don't rush through this process, and be gentle. After all of your hair has been covered with your pre-poo treatment, use the pads of your fingers to gently massage your scalp in a circular motion, moving from your temples to the crown of your head, and down to the nape of your neck.

Once you're finished enjoying your scalp massage, loosely braid each section of your hair and secure the ends gently with the same scrunchie you used before. Now cover your hair with a plastic cap and wait at a few minutes before cleansing your hair. You can also go to sleep with your pre-poo treatment and cleanse hair in the morning. Just make sure to sleep with your plastic cap. You may even want to sleep with an additional head cover. A head cover will help to insulate and gently warm your hair for a deeper conditioning effect while you sleep.

What Should You Use To Pre-Poo?

The pre-poo choice is up to you. During this step, women will typically choose between natural emollients or commercial conditioners, or even infusions with several natural and commercial ingredients. You can use pure coconut oil if you want to keep things simple. Just be sure to gently melt the coconut oil first in a warm bath to allow for easier distribution on hair. Or you can skip the pre-poo step altogether. The choice and use of a pre-poo is not meant to be confusing or complex. If you choose to pre-poo with an emollient, I would advise that you not be heavy-handed. Making your hair extra greasy will create more work for you during the cleansing process. Personally, I like to cleanse my hair once a week. I will share more about Ayurveda and Ayurvedic hair care in a later chapter.

CLEANSING

HOW OFTEN: ONCE A WEEK

Cleansing is done to remove dirt, excess oils and product buildup from your hair. If you don't cleanse your hair regularly, you'll run the risk of dryness as grime accumulates and blocks the hair shaft from absorbing moisture. If that isn't reason enough to regularly cleanse hair, there's also the general unpleasantness of being recognized as the chick with smelly hair, and nobody wants to be *that* chick!

I cleanse my hair once a week. Once a week works for my lifestyle and I don't feel the need to cleanse my hair more often than that. Furthermore, I don't like cleansing more than once a week because it increases the risk of altering the acid mantle of my hair and scalp, stripping natural oils from my hair, and ultimately increasing the damage done to my hair as a result of more manipulation.

For the cleansing step I typically use a commercial conditioner. Yes, you can use a conditioner to cleanse your hair! This is called co-washing. If you've never heard of co-washing, I'll give you a quick run-down.

Funny thing is a male friend overheard a small snippet of conversation about co-washing. He instantly became excited and pulled me aside to learn more. It truly disappointed him to learn that co-washing didn't mean women taking showers together.

Co-washing is simply using conditioner to cleanse the hair instead of shampoo. So when washing your hair, you simply cut out the shampoo step and go straight to conditioning. Although it may seem weird to use a conditioner instead of shampoo, the fact is that conditioners are just as effective for cleansing hair. This is because most conditioners already have cleansing agents as ingredients. Furthermore, conditioners are typically less harsh, more moisturizing, and have reconstructing capabilities that shampoos lack. I'm not totally knocking shampoo because it is fine for cleansing hair. However, if you haven't done so already, you should switch to sulfate-free shampoos immediately. As I explained earlier, sulfates are cleansing agents that are included in most commercial shampoos. Sulfates are what give shampoos their bubbly, foamy quality. Sulfates may make bath time fun, but they are also powerful degreasers that will literally strip the oil from your hair- and you don't want that!

Personally, I've found that co-washing is a wonderful alternative to shampoo. Basically, I look at co-washing as an excellent means to condition and cleanse my hair. It's like getting two benefits for the price of one.

If you choose to co-wash, you can use any type of commercial conditioner you'd like. However, I should point out that there are drawbacks to co-washing. The biggest drawback is product buildup, most often due to silicones. This issue becomes even more common in areas with hard water.

Silicones are agents that give hair "slip" and shine. Silicones are frequently added to commercial conditioners and come in two forms: water-soluble and non-water-soluble. Water soluble silicones rinse easily from hair, while non-water-soluble silicones cannot be easily washed from hair without the use of an acid rinse or a stronger cleansing agent, like a shampoo containing sulfates. By the way, "clarifying shampoos" are simply shampoos with sulfates.

When silicone isn't regularly cleansed from hair, you will run the risk of silicone and product buildup. To help avoid the silicone and product buildup dilemma, it may be best to select those conditioners with water-soluble silicones (or even a silicone-free conditioner if that's what you'd like). This means you will need to read the labels on commercial conditioners. Silicones can be easily identified by looking for words with these endings: *-cone, -conol, -col* and *-xane.*

To tell if your conditioner contains water-soluble silicones, just read the ingredients on the bottle and look for silicones with "PEG" or "PPG" in front of the name. Silicones that are also soluble in water, but not listed with PEG/PPG in front of them, include: Dimethicone Copolyol, Hydroxypropyl Polysiloxane and Lauryl methicone copolyol. If your conditioner contains these silicones, then you will not have an issue with product buildup.

A few *slightly* water-soluble and non-water-soluble silicones include: Amodimethicone, Behenoxy Dimethicone, Cetearyl Methicone, Cetyl Dimethicone, Cyclomethicone, Cyclopentasiloxane, Dimethicone, Dimethiconol, Phenyl Trimethicone, Polydimethysiloxane, Simethicone, Stearyl Dimethicone, Trimethicone, Trimethylsilylamodimethicone. If your conditioner contains these types of silicones product buildup may become an issue if you don't regularly clarify your hair.

If you just took a minute to examine your current conditioner bottle and realized that it does not contain water-soluble silicones, don't worry about the cost of finding those that do. There are tons of low cost conditioners that contain water-soluble silicones or no silicones at all. You won't have to break your piggy bank when looking for a great conditioner for co-washing.

How Often Should You Co-wash?
Once again, cleansing frequency is all personal preference. You can keep your current regimen, while simply eliminating the shampoo step. If you

normally wash your hair twice a week, you can transition to co-washing your hair twice a week. It's really up to you. But, if you do decide to co-wash frequently I would strongly suggest using products with water-soluble silicones. Even though I tend to cleanse my hair once a week, I try to use conditioners that contain only water-soluble silicones. I do this because I want to minimize the risk of product buildup. If at any time I feel like my hair is becoming dull, weighed down, or suffering from product buildup, I simply clarify my hair with a sulfate-free shampoo or an apple cider vinegar rinse. Once again, I don't use acid rinses or shampoos more often than once a month. I find that a monthly clarifying treatment is all my hair needs.

APPLE CIDER VINEGAR RINSE (ACV RINSE)

Ingredients: 2 cups of water (bottled/filtered water), 2 Tsp. apple cider vinegar (Braggs Organic Apple Cider Vinegar)

Directions: Mix ingredients in an applicator bottle. Squeeze over hair while massaging scalp and lightly scrunching hair to remove buildup. Acid rinses are used as a final rinse for hair to help restore pH balance and seal the cuticle. *Do not use undiluted ACV on hair.*

HOW TO CLEANSE

When cleansing long hair, it's best to keep hair in the same braids that were made during the pre-poo step. This will reduce the likelihood of tangling. Sometimes braids will come loose while cleansing. If this happens, just pause for a minute to re-braid your hair, then resume with cleansing. Here are the steps for cleansing your hair:

1. Adjust the water temperature to warm.

2. Tilt your head back into the water and allow the water to fully soak your hair. Do not scrub or rub your hair.

3. If you're co-washing, generously coat your hair with conditioner in a smoothing down motion. If you're using shampoo, first apply shampoo to your fingertips and gently massage your cleanser *directly onto your scalp*, not your hair. This is important. If you use shampoo during the cleansing step, you want to focus on only shampooing your scalp, not your hair. Remember, shampoo can have a drying effect on hair. After you've applied cleanser, massage your scalp in a gentle, circular motion from the front of your scalp to the crown of your head, and ending at the nape of your neck. When massaging your scalp, allow hair to move gently between your fingers. Allow your hair to fall naturally as you work your fingers through your hair. Don't manipulate your hair more than necessary. Don't pile hair on top of your head as you massage, and don't rub or scrub the ends of your hair.

4. Tilt your head back into the stream of water from your showerhead and allow the water to thoroughly rinse through your hair. The run-off from your cleanser coupled with the pressure of the water will be enough to cleanse the ends of your hair. If you feel like you need a little extra help cleansing the ends of your hair, you can use your hands to do a gentle cupping and squeezing motion around your braids. This will help push water through your hair and help with cleansing. A cupping and gentle squeezing motion is all that's needed. Do not scrub your hair.

5. If you feel like your hair needs an extra cleanse, repeat steps three and four. Be mindful about over-cleansing your hair (especially if you're using a shampoo). You want to cleanse your hair, but you don't want to risk stripping the natural oil from your hair.

6. On the final rinse you should unbraid your hair and use cool or the coldest water you can bear. Cool water will help to flatten cuticles and seal the hair. As cool water rinses through your hair, you can gently comb your fingers through your hair to remove any tangles.

While doing this you may notice a few shed hairs on your fingers. This is perfectly normal, as the average person can shed up to 200 hairs per wash.

7. Once you've finished rinsing, use your hands to gently squeeze excess water from your hair.

8. After squeezing excess water from your hair, gently pat your hair dry with a soft cotton t-shirt or microfiber towel. When drying your hair, use a patting motion. Do not vigorously rub your hair and do not use a conventional towel to dry your hair. The fibers in conventional towels are too rough and will absorb too much moisture from your hair.

DEEP CONDITIONING

HOW OFTEN: ONCE A WEEK FOR MOISTURIZING TREATMENTS AND ONCE EVERY SIX WEEKS FOR PROTEIN TREATMENTS

Deep conditioning gives back to hair what time and damage has taken away- moisture and protein. Deep conditioners can fall into two categories: moisturizing deep conditioners that aim to give hair more moisture, or heavier protein-based deep conditioners that serve to only reconstruct hair. In reality, most commercial conditioners contain ingredients to dually moisturize and reconstruct hair. Remember, most commercial conditioners already contain proteins, most often "lighter" proteins. Thus, many commercial conditioners can be used as deep conditioners. In fact, countless commercial conditioners already contain many of the same ingredients that are used in products that are packaged as "deep conditioners." The only difference is that the "deep conditioner" was simply packaged differently and oftentimes priced higher. For this very reason, I let my co-wash conditioner serve as a cleanser and as a moisturizing deep conditioning treatment. If you shampoo your hair, you should most certainly follow up with a conditioner or deep conditioner. In some cases women also like to use a different deep conditioner product after every co-wash. That's not something I typically do, although I do like to use a more intense, deep conditioner (like a protein treatment) once every 4-6 weeks.

How Long Should You Deep Condition?

I've noticed that there's a considerably broad range of time frames that women will deep condition their hair. For example, I know many women who are fans of deep conditioning treatments that can last from 30 minutes and up to 60 minutes. Then, there are some women who like to deep condition their hair overnight. How long you choose to deep condition is up to you.

I've heard all the debate and questions about whether deep conditioning is a myth and how long you should deep condition. I don't concern myself too much with it. Overall, I'm a big advocate of going with what makes me and my hair feel good. Personally, I've found that 10-15 minutes is sufficient time for my conditioner treatment to work. That's just how I do it and I don't find longer times necessary in most cases.

Do You Need Heat To Deep Condition?

It's a common misconception that you should always use heat for deep conditioning. If a conditioner is meant to be used with heat, the manufacturer's instructions will explicitly tell you to apply heat for a specific amount of time. Not every conditioner is meant to be used with heat. Yes, heat will help to raise the cuticle and allow for deeper conditioner penetration into the hair shaft. But heat will only increase the effect of a conditioner if it has been formulated with penetrating ingredients that require heat. Furthermore, it's not necessarily an issue of conditioners that require heat working better than conditioners that are simply rinsed from hair after a few minutes.

The conditioners I currently use don't require heat and I think they work fine. If you want to use heat to deep condition, feel free to do so, but realize that it may not always be necessary. The overall effect of a conditioner ultimately depends on the ingredients of the conditioner, as well as whether you properly use the conditioner as instructed by the manufacturer.

MOISTURIZING

HOW OFTEN: DAILY

Moisture will help to counteract the natural dryness of afro-textured hair. Our hair loves moisture. So, I make sure to moisturize my hair twice a day in two different ways. In the morning, I shower with my hair uncovered and let the steam from my shower moisturize my hair. Remember, water is the ultimate moisturizer. Steam from my shower works just fine for moisturizing my hair in the morning. Then, later on in the evening, I'll also lightly spray my hair with a homemade moisturizing spray that contains ingredients like aloe vera, vegetable glycerin and/or marshmallow root. On other evenings I may choose to use a moisturizing spray that contains a mix of one part curl activator spray, one part distilled water, and a few drops of essential oil. This is just the way I do it, but you can set up your moisturizing regimen however you want. Just remember to moisturize your hair daily.

HOW TO MOISTURIZE

Keep your moisturizer stored in a spray bottle that gives off a wide, even mist when sprayed. When moisturizing, spray all of your hair while concentrating on the ends. You do not need to saturate your hair with moisturizer. You're not going for the curl activator, *Soul-Glo* look. Just lightly mist your hair. Then use your fingers to gently detangle hair. The slip from your moisturizing spray will help loosen any tangles.

MOISTURIZING SPRITZ

Ingredients: 12 ounces distilled water, 1-2 tablespoons of vegetable glycerin

Directions: Combine ingredients in spray bottle. Shake well. Spritz as needed. You can also add a few drops of your favorite essential oil(s) to this spritz. When using homemade moisturizers with natural humectants like vegetable glycerin, it's important to sufficiently dilute in water first before using on hair. Natural humectants are syrupy in consistency and tend to be sticky. If not diluted properly, they can also make hair sticky.

SEALING

HOW OFTEN: EVERY DAY AFTER MOISTURIZING

After moisturizing your hair, you should always seal in the moisture with an emollient. Sealing hair is important because without it, hair would simply lose moisture through evaporation. This step is especially important for women with highly porous hair. As far as sealant options go, you can use whatever you want. I prefer natural emollients.

HOW TO SEAL

Gently rub your favorite emollient in the palm of your hands. Evenly distribute the oil to your hair, smoothing from root to tip. You do not need to be heavy-handed with the amount of emollient you use. Applying too much will weigh hair down. This is why I like to use light butters and oils for sealing. A helpful trick is to add your favorite oil(s) to a spray bottle. Then use this bottle to *lightly* mist hair. After misting hair, gently smooth down hair from root to tip. The smoothing down motion will help to seal in moisture, flatten the cuticle and add sheen. I really like the spray bottle method for sealing my hair.

STIMULATING

HOW OFTEN: ONCE A DAY

Stimulating involves gently massaging the scalp with an oil or oil infusion. This is the step where you really want to focus on relaxation. Scalp massages help relieve tension and trigger the release of feel-good hormones like dopamine and serotonin. Scalp massages also stimulate blood flow to the hair follicles. Blood flow to hair follicles is vital for hair growth. I give myself scalp massages almost daily for a couple of minutes at a time. I usually do them right after I've finished applying a seal to my hair. I simply use the same oil I used to seal my hair or I'll use an emollient blended with ingredients like peppermint, rosemary, and clary sage oil.

HOW TO STIMULATE

When stimulating your scalp, place oil on your fingertips and massage your scalp with the pads of your fingers in a gentle circular motion. Move your fingers from your temples to the crown of your head and then finally to the nape of your neck. You may also want to gently massage your shoulders since many of us carry tension there. Take your time during this step and relax.

PROTECTIVE STYLING

HOW OFTEN: ALMOST DAILY

Protective styling is the last step of my *labor of love*. As previously explained, afro-textured hair is more delicate and more prone to damage than other hair types. For this very reason, I believe protective styling is an absolute must for growing hair to longer lengths. Protectively styling your hair will help you achieve longer length by 1) eliminating or reducing breakage and 2) eliminating or reducing the frequency of knotting and tangling.

A protective style is achieved when individual strands of hair are not worn free-flowing and loose. The ends of the hair are either tucked away or worn off the shoulders. This is done to protect the ends of your hair, which are also the oldest and most fragile part of your hair. Protective styles can be worn for multiple days at a time, eliminating the need to frequently manipulate hair. Common protective styles include french rolls, cornrows, buns, braids, twists, and even weaves or wigs. Basically, any style that tucks away your hair and reduces the need to frequently manipulate it is a protective style.

My hair is protectively styled almost daily in two-strand twists. On special occasions I do like to unravel my twists, fluff my hair, and rock my big ole 'fro. If I'm too tired to re-twist my hair before bed I'll make sure to loosely braid my hair in large plaits or wear it in a high ponytail at the crown of my head before going to sleep. This high ponytail is often called "pineappling" or a samurai bun. I also make sure to cover my hair every night with a satin bonnet for protection. Overall, I have a very protective hair regimen, and this is what has enabled me to achieve length. Protection is what your hair needs to grow. Remember, you always protect what you love.

TAKE HOME POINTS

My hair regimen breaks down into seven steps: pre-cleansing, cleansing, deep conditioning, moisturizing, sealing, stimulating, and protective styling.

My pre-poo treatment consists of lightly coating the hair with a natural emollient or an Ayurvedic treatment before every wash.

A cleansing and moisturizing deep conditioning is done once a week and consists of co-washing with 1) a conditioner that contains water-soluble silicones or 2) a silicone-free conditioner. (Hair is also "clarified" with an acid rinse or a sulfate-free shampoo once a month if necessary).

An additional deep conditioning is done once every six weeks with a protein treatment.

Moisturizing is done twice-daily with a water-based moisturizer, and hair is sealed afterward with a natural emollient.

Scalp massages are regularly performed and protective styles are worm almost daily.

Hair is covered with a satin bonnet every night.

CHAPTER 11
SEASONAL HAIR TIPS

One of the coolest things about living in DC is that I get to experience all of the seasons. During the summer I can take a short trip to the beach to soak up the sun. During the winter I can play in the snow while rocking cute boots and overcoats. I also make sure to enjoy all the fabulous weather in between. But, while seasonal change can be tons of fun, it can also present a few challenges for my hair. I tend to tweak my hair regimen based on the weather because some things that work really well for my hair in the summer may not work as well during the winter. Overall, it's a smart move to be flexible with your hair regimen and adapt to the seasons. You never want to be too rigid because you could end up counteracting your growth potential. Here are a few suggestions to help you and your hair navigate all four seasons:

SPRING & SUMMER

During the spring/summer months, the most common things to worry about are UVA/UVB ray exposure, humidity and harsh water exposure from the beach and chlorinated pools.

SUN DAMAGE

Hair can get damaged from UV rays all year round, but the risk of damage is even greater in the spring and summer months, since we're more likely to be outdoors with our heads uncovered for longer periods of time. We constantly hear about using sunscreen for our skin, but sun rays can be just as damaging to our hair. Sun rays can fade hair color, weaken the hair shaft, and cause split ends. Plus, heat from the sun is also very drying and can literally bake moisture right out of the hair shaft.

To protect hair from prolonged sun exposure you should do three very basic things:

1. Wear a head covering

2. Use hair products with sunscreen.

3. Carry a travel-size spray bottle of moisturizer to use on hair throughout the day

When using head coverings make sure to use those that have an inner lining made of soft silk-like material. As for hair products, there are many natural emollients that offer excellent UV-ray protection. There are also many commercial products that are manufactured with added sunscreen.

HUMIDITY

Humidity is a term used to describe the amount of water vapor (i.e. moisture) in the air. High humidity levels tend to make our hair and body feel sticky. People do tend to perceive humidity differently, so to gauge humidity in more absolute terms, you can look at the *dew point*. When you check the weather for the day, look for the dew point. The dew point is basically the temperature at which air is saturated with water. The higher the dew point, the more moisture will be in the air. In simplest terms, the higher the dew point, the more humid air will feel. At dew points above 65°F, air tends to feel sticky and humid. Air is often perceived as comfortable and moderate at dew points between 50°F and 60°F. Lastly, at dew points less than 49°F, air as perceived as more dry and desert-like.

In dew points above 65°F, humidity can present a few problems for hair (especially porous hair). Hair has the ability to act like a sponge and literally drink moisture from the air. When this happens, the hair shaft will become swollen, the cuticles will rise, and you'll end up with hair that's frizzy and prone to tangling.

You want to keep hair moisturized regardless of the dew point, but you need to be careful when using humectants in high and low dew point temperatures. While humectants can be great for locking in moisture in moderate climates, at high dew points, humectants can draw in more moisture from the air and exacerbate the effects of humidity. Furthermore, at very low dew points, humectants can actually have the opposite effect and pull moisture away from the hair, causing dryness. Remember, humectants simply pull water from one area to another. *Humectants don't always moisturize hair.* Because of this effect, it has been recommended that women with afro-textured hair consider using humectants at dew points between 35°F and 50°F. And if you choose to use humectants at higher dew point temperatures (i.e. 60°F or above), it would be wise to also effectively seal your hair with an emollient (which are sometimes called anti-humectants). In cases of high humidity, this seal will block the humectant from pulling in too much moisture into the hair shaft.

SWIMMER'S HAIR

Not all water will have a moisturizing effect on hair. In fact certain types of water, like salt water from the beach and chlorinated water from swimming pools, can be very harsh and have a drying effect on hair.

If you're like me and literally live in the water during the summer months, you will want to take extra precautions against harsh water. The best ways to do this are by following these steps:

1. Wear a protective style before getting in the water.

2. Do not cleanse your hair before getting in the water. The natural oils and product buildup on your hair and scalp will actually serve as a protective barrier against harsh water.

3. Instead of cleansing your hair, simply rinse your hair with fresh water. The fresh water will help to saturate your hair and prevent absorption of salt or chlorine water into the hair shaft.

4. After rinsing your hair with fresh water, thoroughly coat your hair with a natural emollient. This will lock moisture in and work to form a barrier to further block out harsh water. One easy trick is to fill a spray bottle with your favorite natural oil, then mist your hair.

5. Consider wearing a swimmers cap instead of leaving hair uncovered. I know, I know. It doesn't look as sexy as a Bond girl style exit from the water, but a swimmer's cap will definitely help to keep your hair protected from harsh water. Swimmers caps can fit pretty snug, so before putting one on you may want to spray the inner lining of the cap with oil. This will make it easier to slide the cap on and off your head.

6. Next, splash around and have fun!

7. Once you're out of the water, immediately and thoroughly rinse your hair with fresh water. Then follow up with a leave-in conditioner.

FALL & WINTER

Though the fall and winter months tend to present fewer complications for hair, these months can still present a few unique hair challenges. The biggest of these challenges is chronic dry hair due to cool, low humidity air. The hot sun from the summer is no longer baking moisture out of your hair, but during the drier winter months, low humidity air can also work to leech moisture from your hair. Here are a few tips to keep hair moisturized and well-conditioned during the fall and winter months:

GET A HUMIDIFIER

Cold air tends to have less moisture, and this moisture is further decreased when we run our heaters and use fireplaces. If my hair had to choose between living in humid air or dry air, it would choose humid every time. I prefer environments where my hair is surrounded by an abundance of moisture. Dry air and dry climates pull moisture from hair. So as far as I'm concerned, a humidifier is a must during the winter months. Humidifiers will replace moisture in the air and help to keep hair (and skin) from becoming overly dry.

USE A STRONGER SEAL

You should regularly moisturize and seal your hair regardless of the time of year. However, during the colder (and drier) months you may also want to consider using a heavier emollient to form a better seal and prevent moisture loss from hair. During the late fall and winter months, lighter emollients may be a bit less effective in preventing moisture loss. That is why I like to use heavier emollients like shea butter and castor oil during this time of year. Everyone's hair is different, but I know my hair thrives with a lighter emollient in the warmer months and a heavier emollient in the colder months.

USE HAIR FRIENDLY HATS AND HEAD COVERS

One of the things I love about fall and winter is fashion. During this time of the year I always go on a mini shopping spree for a variety of winter hats and knit caps. But while I do love stocking up on super cute head gear, I'm also mindful of avoiding those that are made of material that can damage the cuticle or pull moisture from the hair shaft. If you like to wear winter hats and knit caps (especially those made of cotton or yarn-like fabric),

I would urge you to look for covers that are made with smooth, silk or stain-like inner linings. And if your head gear doesn't have this type of lining, it's not that hard to buy the material and sew one in yourself.

CLEANSE LESS OFTEN

Practically speaking, you should not wash your hair frequently during the cold, drier months. Washing hair frequently will accelerate damage and increase the likelihood of removing natural oils from the hair and scalp. Furthermore, the already cold, dry winter air will further exacerbate moisture loss from the hair shaft, which could ultimately lead to breakage. This is why I especially don't wash my hair more than once a week during the fall/winter months. You can wash your hair as often as you would like, but during colder months I strongly advise against washing hair frequently.

BE CAREFUL WITH HUMECTANT USE

As mentioned earlier, humectants can actually work against hair in areas of very low humidity. During the winter (and in dew points less than 35°F), humectants can actually work to pull moisture from the hair. Because of this, I tend to stay away from humectants during the winter. Some women like to use humectants, regardless of the weather, and if you plan on using a humectant during the winter, pay very close attention to how well your hair is moisturized during the day. If you notice drier hair, fly-aways, split ends, and broken strands, then you may want to discontinue using humectants until the temperature and dew point become more agreeable.

TAKE HOME POINTS

Be mindful about keeping hair moisturized, regardless of the time of year.

Take precautions against harsh water (i.e. salt water from the beach and chlorinated water from swimming pools) during summer months.

Wear hair friendly head covers that won't rob your hair of moisture or cause friction against the hair shaft.

During the colder months consider using a heavier emollient to form a better seal and prevent moisture loss from hair.

Consider washing hair less often during the winter months.

Be careful with humectant use. Humectants are used as moisturizers, but they simply work by pulling water from one area to another. Under certain temperature conditions, humectants can have a negative moisturizing effect on hair. Because of this negative effect, it has been recommended that women with afro-textured hair consider using humectants at dew points between 35°-50°F.

CHAPTER 12

TRIMMING HAIR

The frequency in which you trim your hair is a very important factor to consider if you're attempting to grow longer hair. Some women avoid trimming their hair as much as possible, while others see frequent trims as essential for hair growth. On the topic, I sit firmly in on the grounds of *trim as needed*. I certainly don't advocate pointless trims, but I do know that trimming is useful for the appearance of healthy hair growth.

I know many women that hate trimming their hair and tense up whenever they see a stylist coming near them with a pair of scissors. I do recognize that there are a few stylists that may be a bit too "trim-happy" and advocate pointless hair trimming. Then there are also folks spreading the myth that trimming your hair will make it grow faster or longer. I'm sorry to break the news but that myth is absolutely false.

Make no mistake, trimming *should* be a regular part of hair maintenance, but it will not make your hair grow. As far as trimming hair goes, if your goals are length *and* a healthy appearance, you will need to pay attention to 3 key factors:

Factor #1 - How protective you are with your hair

Factor #2 - The *amount* of hair you trim at a time

Factor #3 - The *frequency* at which you trim your hair

When hair grows, it will reach a critical length where the cuticle becomes worn away from chronic damage. At this critical length, the ends of the hair will taper, and the cortex may even be completely exposed. This is usually the point where the ends of the hair will start to look jagged and less full. You want to trim away these ends because the cuticle is no longer present for protection. You also want to trim this part away because it will start to make the rest of your hair look less appealing or healthy. This critical length will happen in everyone's hair, just at different lengths. It's an inescapable fact that the ends of your hair, which are also the oldest part of your hair, will naturally become more and more damaged as time progresses. Furthermore, you can speed up the appearance of this critical length if you frequently damage your hair.

On average, I only trim my hair every six months or so, by performing a light "dusting" of my ends (i.e. removing split ends as I see them). I can trim this way because I control the rate of damage by being protective with my hair. This is another big reason why I treat my hair the way I do; it cuts down on the need to frequently trim my ends. Women who are very protective with their hair will not need to frequently trim their ends. Women who are less protective with their hair will need to trim more often. It's as simple as that.

Just accept that you can't run from trims entirely, no matter how protective you are with your hair. In every case, there is a critical length where hair will become so damaged that it needs to be trimmed. Knowing this, it makes sense to be as protective as possible so that your critical length takes longer to appear. How much and how often you need to trim your hair is going to be dependent on how well you take care of your hair.

In addition to taking care of your hair, one other factor that you should also be aware of before trimming hair is the natural occurrence of uneven hair growth. All of your hair follicles are not working in perfect unison when producing hair. Some hair follicles will be in an active growing phase while other hair follicles will be in the transition or resting phase.

As a result, you will experience hair that appears to grow faster or longer at a particular part of your scalp. When this happens the ends of your hair will look slightly uneven, and could even be mistaken for hair that needs to be trimmed because it is suffering from damage or breakage.

Don't worry if you're maintaining a protective hair regimen but notice that the ends of your hair look uneven over time. What you're observing is simply uneven hair growth which is perfectly natural and very common. That stated, if you're trying to grow your hair out, you shouldn't obsessively trim the ends of your hair every time it looks uneven. In fact, if you know for certain that your hair is growing unevenly, you can wait a few weeks for the shorter part of your hair to catch up before trimming. Uneven ends don't always mean "damaged ends." So while you should make sure to regularly trim away the damaged ends of your hair, you don't always have to immediately trim your hair simply because it looks uneven.

Ultimately, if you are interested in growing longer hair, you should take care of your hair and trim it less than the rate at which your hair grows. For example, if your hair grows half an inch per month, you don't want to trim off an inch of hair every month. The best thing to do would be to trim an inch every three, four or even six months. Trimming can be done by you, a friend or a professional stylist. When trimming your own ends you should use a quality pair of hair scissors that are sharp and only used for cutting hair. Set your own schedule for trimming. If you maintain a protective hair regimen, you won't need to make large or frequent cuts.

TAKE HOME POINTS

The ends of hair will naturally become damaged as time goes on. The extent of damage is controlled by how protective you are with your hair.

As hair grows, it will reach a critical length where the ends have cuticles that have worn away from chronic damage. You want to trim away these ends because the cuticle is no longer present for protection.

Women who are very protective with their hair will be able to grow hair longer and faster because they will not need to frequently trim hair to remove damaged ends.

Uneven hair growth is a natural and common occurrence. In order to grow hair to longer lengths, hair should not be trimmed simply because it looks uneven.

CHAPTER 13
AYURVEDA

By this point in the book you should fully understand the importance of approaching hair growth from a more holistic standpoint that includes a healthy diet, exercise, and even stress management. And now I want to talk a little more in-depth about a type of holistic, healthy living practice called Ayurveda. For those new to the subject of Ayurveda, the word itself translates to "the complete knowledge for long life" and many scholars consider Ayurveda to be one of the oldest healing sciences. Ayurveda is also a form of alternative medicine that can be practiced by anyone because the principles are universal and based on the laws and cycles of Mother Nature.

In a nutshell, Ayurveda teaches that everything in the universe is made of five elements: space, air, fire, water, and earth. So, everything in the world (including you) is made up of one, two, or a more complex combination of these five elements. Any change that occurs within us and the world is simply a change from one element to another. Furthermore, Ayurveda also teaches us that beauty is not a superficial, solitary attribute. Instead true beauty is defined by three key attributes:

Outer beauty - defined by the appearance of the skin and hair

Inner beauty - defined by clarity of the mind and confidence

Lasting beauty - defined by the ability to exude health and beauty throughout life

BALANCE FOR HEALTH & BEAUTY

Overall Ayurveda teaches that in order to achieve beauty and harmony, a person must have balance in their life. Imbalances can be caused by things like poor diet, lack of exercise, inadequate rest, stress, and even repressed emotions, like anger or resentment, can cause imbalance. And ultimately Ayurveda teaches us that in order to avoid disease, dysfunction, and even hair loss, we need to do our best to lead more healthy, balanced lifestyles.

AYURVEDIC HAIR CARE

The reason why I wanted to share a little bit about Ayurveda is because it's an interesting topic and healing science that has become increasingly popular in beauty and the hair care industry, and quite a few aspects of my lifestyle and haircare regimen naturally follow principles of Ayurvea. So within Ayurveda there are many Ayurvedic herbs and oils can be used to cleanse, condition and strengthen hair. They can also be used to color hair, and some treatments can be used to cure scalp ailments. In addition to that, Ayurveda also encourages women to avoid chemical-based hair care and heat styling, as well as less than healthy hair care practices that can cause hair damage and even health complications in the long term.

All the above understood, if you're looking more natural hair care products to incorporate into your regimen, you may want to look into Ayurvedic products, and in this chapter I have included a list of Ayurvedic herbs and oils that may be beneficial to healthy hair growth. These herbs and oils are typically used as herbal cleansers, conditioners and/or hair oils. Also, many of the herbs are frequently sold as powders that are then blended with water and made into a thick paste before they are applied to the scalp and hair.

Before using any Ayurvedic product or treatment, here are a few useful tips:

1. Always perform a skin test to make sure you're not allergic. Certain herbs and oils may cause slight darkening or reddening of hair, especially when left on hair for long periods of time. You may want to first test pastes on shed hair to early detect any color changes. You should always use plastic/glass bowls as well as plastic utensils when mixing pastes. Never use metal containers or metal utensils. You should also have gloves, a plastic cap, and an applicator brush handy for use.

2. Before using an Ayurvedic herb or oil, it's best to first define what results you want with your hair, and then pick your products accordingly. Mixing is not an exact science and you will have to figure out what works for you. You can also add herbs and oils to your commercial products. All in all, making your own haircare treatments should be simple and stress-free. If you are a newbie to this, try not to overdue things by mixing too many ingredients and overwhelming yourself. Remember, the goal is to establish your own healthy hair care regimen, not lose all your hair from stressing yourself out.

3. Since herbs do have a shelf-life, it is always best to buy reasonable amounts at a time and store any unused packages of herb in airtight plastic or glass containers. When making your pastes, I would suggest that you keep a journal of ingredients and results. This will help you to repeat and duplicate the results that you like. Finally, I'd also advise taking pictures of your hair before and after a treatment. This way you can keep a digital journal of your hair's progress.

4. All of the herbs and oils listed in this chapter can be found via online distributors like Amazon, as well as at your local Indian market. Whenever you decide to buy always make sure they are a reputable distributor

Overall, Ayurvedic haircare can be as simple or as complicated as you want to make it. Some Ayurvedic products are sold as a simple pure herb or oil, and some products, such as Kalpi Tone and Ayurvedic shampoo bars, already come as an infusion of several Ayurvedic herbs and oils. So what you'll need to do is first determine the condition of your hair and what you'd like to achieve. In the next section of this chapter I have listed a few popular Ayurvedic herbs and oils. Keep in mind that I haven't used all of these Ayurvedic products, and I'm not saying that you need to either. Overall, the following information is meant to be a reference source for women who want to learn a bit more about natural products that they can use for haircare. And ultimately, whether you choice to use Ayurvedic or other natural haircare products is totally up to you..

AMLA

Known for its rich content of vitamin C, amla is used for conditioning, strengthening, boosting sheen, preventing premature graying and ppromting healthy hair growth. Amla can be mixed with water or aloe gel to make a hair conditioning paste. Amla also blends well with shikakai, aritha, neem and/or bhringraj powders.

AMLA OIL

Amla oil has many of the same benefits as the powder. It is sold as the pure oil itself and as an infusion with other herbs and ingredients. Amla oil can be used daily to oil the scalp and seal the hair.

ARGAN OIL

Argan oil is rich in vitamin E, omega-6 essential fatty acids, and is a popular ingredient in commercial hair products. Moroccan oil is another name for argan oil. *Moroccan oil* is sometimes referred to as "liquid gold," and is extracted from the fruit of Argan trees found predominately in Morocco. This oil can be added to deep conditioning treatments. It can also be used on the hair and scalp daily.

ARITHA/REETHA

Aritha is commonly referred to as "soapnut" and is a popular ingredient in Ayurvedic shampoos and cleansers. It is used to prevent dandruff and also has insecticidal abilities. Aritha can be somewhat drying and may leave hair feeling a bit stiff. Before using you may want to mix it in an applicator bottle with water. Use the applicator bottle to pour cleansing solution directly onto the scalp (not to hair). Mixing aritha with conditioning herbs like amla or hibiscus can counteract its drying effect. It is best to avoid mixing aritha with shikakai, since both can be drying.

BENTONITE CLAY

Bentonite clay is a mild cleanser, clarifier and detoxifier. Bentonite clay works well when mixed with aloe vera juice or gel. You can use this mixture as a hair-clarifying mask to remove product buildup. When used on afro-textured hair, a bentonite clay mask can help with enhancing curl definition.

BHRINGRAJ

Bhringraj translates to "king of hair." Bhringraj is one of the most popular herbs in Ayurveda. It is frequently used to prevent hair thinning, hair loss, premature graying, dandruff and itchy scalp. Bhringraj also has the ability to slightly darken hair. Bhringraj mixes well with amla, brahmi, shikakai, and/or neem.

BHRINGRAJ OIL

Bhringraj oil has many of the same benefits as the powder. Bhringraj oil can be used as a deep conditioning treatment, or as a simple hair oil for daily use.

BRAHMI

Brahmi is used as a cleanser and conditioner. It is used to strengthen hair roots, prevent hair thinning, hair loss and premature graying. It is also used to treat dandruff and an itchy scalp. Brahmi has the ability to slightly darken hair and mixes will with amla, aritha, bhringraj, shikakai, and/or neem powders.

BRAHMI OIL

Brahmi oil has similar benefits to the powder. It can be purchased in its pure oil form or as an infusion with other exotic Indian herbs. Brahmi oil can be used as a deep conditioning treatment and/or a daily hair oil.

HIBISCUS

Hibiscus is a very versatile herb that is commonly mixed with many other products as a mild cleanser and hair conditioner. Hibiscus contains mucilage, a plant protein that will give hair slip and help with detangling. It also has an abundance of plant proteins that help strengthen and protect hair. It can be added to pre-poos, moisturizers, detanglers, deep conditioners or used in tea rinses. Hibiscus does have the ability to stain porous hair a slight reddish hue.

KALPI TONE

Kalpi Tone is a mix of several herbs. It is used to strengthen the hair shaft and has conditioning properties that give hair softness and sheen. It can also have a slightly darkening effect on hair.

MARSHMALLOW ROOT

Marshmallow root is a very effective detangling agent and conditioner. It is often added to pastes to increase detangling and conditioning properties.

Like hibiscus, this plant is also rich in plant proteins, mucilage, and will give hair incredible sheen.

METHI (FENUGREEK SEED)

Fenugreek seed can be used on the hair and it is also sold as a supplement and can be taken orally to help treat dietary deficiencies such as iron deficiency (which can cause hair loss). Given its historical use for inducing labor, women should use caution when taking fenugreek during pregnancy.

NEEM

Neem is a potent and highly revered herb with many cosmetic and medicinal uses. It also has potent antifungal properties, antibacterial properties, and is used to treat many skin conditions such as acne, lice, dandruff, eczema, psoriasis and an itchy scalp. Neem is very versatile and can be mixed with just about anything.

NEEM OIL

Neem oil has many of the same benefits as the plant. However, the oil can have a stronger, concentrated scent when compared to the plant itself. Because of this, you may want to consider diluting neem oil in a shampoo, conditioner or carrier oil before use.

SHIKAKAI

Shikakai means "fruit for hair" and is used as a cleansing agent and mild conditioner. Shikakai is often an ingredient in herbal shampoos and it can also be used to treat dandruff. For hair that is prone to dryness, shikakai is best used sparingly and mixes well with conditioning herbs like amla and bhringraj.

SHIKAKAI OIL

Shikakai oil has many of the same benefits as the powder. The oil is sold as a pure oil or as an infusion with other natural oils and herbs. Shikakai oil can be used as a pre-poo treatment, in deep conditioners and as a daily hair oil.

VATIKA OIL

Vatika oil is coconut oil infused with many Ayurvedic herbs. The main ingredient, coconut oil, can penetrate the hair shaft, prevent protein loss, and help strengthen hair. Vatika oil is often used as a pre-poo treatment and in deep conditioning treatments.

TAKE HOME POINTS

Ayurveda is a form of alternative medicine and is considered to be one of the oldest healing sciences.

Ayurveda emphasizes that beauty is defined by three key attributes: outer beauty, inner beauty, and lasting beauty.

In order to achieve supreme beauty and health, a person should do their best to live a balanced lifestyle. Imbalances caused by factors like an unhealthy diet, lack of exercise, and stress can lead disease and hair loss.

Ayurveda encourages women to avoid chemical-based hair care and heat styling, as well as other damaging hair care practices that can create hair problems and even health problems in the long term.

A variety of Ayurvedic herbs and oils can be used for cleansing, conditioning and coloring hair.

CHAPTER 14

COLORING HAIR

Coloring your hair is a simple and effective way to enhance your physical appearance and make you stand out from the crowd. But, coloring hair does come with certain drawbacks. For one, there's the damaging effect of chemicals like ammonia and hydrogen peroxide which are commonly used in commercial hair dyes. Commercial dyes containing these types of ingredients will always cause some degree of damage because they end up increasing the porosity and decreasing the elasticity of hair. As a result, using certain commercial coloring options will often leave hair drier, weaker, and more prone to breakage.

There are three main categories of hair coloring options: permanent coloring, semi/demi permanent coloring, and temporary color rinses. Both permanent and semi-permanent colors work by penetrating the cortex layer of the hair. Thus both permanent and semi-permanent coloring can have damaging effects on hair. Permanent coloring is the most damaging to hair because the process will involve some form of exposure to ammonia and/or hydrogen peroxide. But, unlike the other types of coloring options, permanent colors do allow for drastic color changes and near 100% coverage of gray hair. Semi-permanent coloring is not as damaging as permanent coloring, but coloring effects are less vast and not fully guaranteed. Furthermore, with semi-permanent coloring, the color effect will fade after several washes. Finally, temporary rinses are those that deposit color on the cuticle layer of the hair. This type of coloring option is the safest for afro-textured hair. There is no penetration into the cortex, no damage to the hair, and the color effects are generally washed away after ten to fifteen washes.

I've mentioned the damaging effects of agents like peroxide in commercial dyes. But besides all that, it's important to also know that there are health risks associated with long-term exposure to commercial hair dyes containing artificial coloring agents. As a result many health professionals do advise against using commercial hair dyes.

It's scary to think that harmful chemicals are being used in everyday hair dyes, but they are. And ultimately it's your job to arm yourself with as much information as possible, and use that information to choose the healthiest hair care products.

This is a major reason why I have chosen to use as many natural products as possible, and I also choose the most high-quality commercial hair products when possible. Yes, certain high-quality natural and commercial products may cost more, but in the long term it's definitely worth it. I've learned that just because a hair product or treatment is available for use, or even wildly popular among other women, doesn't mean that it is actually safe or healthy for me in the long term. Case in point: commercial hair dyes – which can be quite damaging to hair.

Fortunately, there a few all-natural, plant-derived hair dyes for women like myself who do want the option of coloring their hair without the risk of hair damage or adverse health effects. And once upon a time, way before commercial dyes, women and men were using plant dyes to color and even strengthen their hair. Even today, in many places such as India, the Middle East, and Africa, it's still a very common practice to use plant dyes to color hair. Three very popular plant dyes that can do this are henna, cassia and indigo.

HENNA, CASSIA & INDIGO DYES

Henna, cassia and indigo are all plant-derived products that can alter the hue of hair by depositing color pigments into the hair shaft without the use of harsh, synthetic chemicals, and natural ingredients like espresso coffee, cinnamon, and essential oils can also be added to these types of plant-based coloring treatments in order to boost coloring effects. For example, depending on what it's mixed with, the color you achieve with henna use can range from orange, to auburn, to deep burgundy, to chestnut brown to a rich black.

Keep in mind though that every head of hair is different and there are several factors that determine the dyeing effect of plant dyes. These factors include:

- Your original hair color

- What other natural ingredients you mix with the plant dye

- How long you allow a paste to sit *before* applying to hair

- How long you allow a paste to sit on your hair *during* the dye process

All the above understood, it's important to follow directions closely when using plant dyes- especially if you are attempting this process by yourself. For example, some venders sell variable forms of henna, often called "compound henna." These types of henna are not pure and are usually blended with metallic dyes and other chemicals. Using compound henna can severely damage your hair and you should not use this form of henna. You should only use BAQ henna (Body Art Quality), which is a high-grade form of henna. BAQ henna can be safely used on all hair types, whether hair is natural or processed.

One more thing – if you plan on using plant dyes to color your hair, be prepared to invest a little time, because plant dyes like henna, cassia and indigo do require a bit more time to mix and prepare when compared to commercial dyes. Even still, there are many people who love using plant dyes like henna to both color and condition their hair, which is something that a commercial dye containing harsh chemicals will never do.

GRAY HAIR

Gray hair is a normal part of aging. Each hair follicle that you have contains a set number of pigment cells that produce *melanin*, the substance that gives hair its natural color. When hair is growing, hair follicle cells and pigment cells work together to produce colored hair. However, as you get older, pigment cells will stop producing as much melanin. At this point hair will then start to lose its color and appear gray. In fact, gray hair is not really gray at all. Your hair and nails are made of the same colorless protein- keratin. Without the staining of melanin from pigment cells, your hair will become colorless just like your fingernails. So, gray hair is really transparent or colorless. It just looks gray due to an optical illusion!

While gray hair is a natural occurrence, premature graying can be brought on by hormonal imbalances and deficiencies in certain nutrients. For example, a deficiency in vitamin B12 can lead to premature graying. An imbalance in thyroid hormone can also cause premature graying. Some people even say that premature graying can be brought on by stress.

THE BEAUTY IN EMBRACING GRAY HAIR

Gray hair, or silver hair as some call it, is just a normal part of life. But as women age, it does become a bit harder for some of us to fully embrace our new silver strands. With men, graying hair is often seen as a sign of maturity, almost like a fine wine getting better with age. This isn't the case with women. Oftentimes, social stigma and double standards can lead many women to buy into the false notion that their silver strands are something to be ashamed of. As a result, it's not uncommon for women to seek hair coloring as a way to "preserve" their appearance of youth.

Despite what society or insecurity tells us, it's important to realize that gray hair is not something to be embarrassed over, nor is it a sign of lost youth or attractiveness. Gray hair is natural *and* it's beautiful- just as beautiful as any other color. Furthermore, beauty is all about attitude and confidence. And many would argue that there is something incredibly beautiful and alluring about a woman who has the confidence to embrace aging and her graying hair, rather than hide from it.

TAKE HOME POINTS

Coloring your hair with commercial dyes will result in variable degrees of hair damage. Commercial dyes may also contain artificial agents that carry long-term health risks.

Coloring hair with plant dyes such as henna, cassia and indigo are more natural alternatives to using commercial hair dyes that may contain harsh chemicals.

Always purchase henna, cassia and indigo dyes from reputable distributors. Henna can be used to dually deep condition and color treat hair. You should only use BAQ henna (Body Art Quality) on hair.

Gray hair is a normal part of aging and is the result of pigment cells that stop producing melanin. Premature graying can also occur due to hormonal imbalances and deficiencies in certain nutrients, such as vitamin B12.

CHAPTER 15
TRUSTING OTHERS WITH YOUR HAIR

I remember when I first moved to the Washington, D.C. area and spent weeks looking for a new stylist and salon. I just wanted a professional place I could go to for an occasional trim or treatment. I wasn't looking for anything extraordinary, just simple hair maintenance, and of course the typical girl chatter and networking that goes hand in hand with getting your hair done.

By this time I had become very educated about my hair and had developed a certain standard that I expected from my hair stylist. Basically, I expected that he/she be respectful and very knowledgeable about hair care. I also wanted someone who would understand my hair goals and help me to achieve them in the best way possible.

During my search for a new stylist I did come across a few that wanted to do things to my hair that were completely contrary to its health. For example, when I explained that I wanted a trim, several stylists insisted on washing my hair first, then blow-drying it, and then flat ironing it straight before they would trim my ends. I tried to convince them that it wasn't necessary to apply so much heat to my hair before a trim, but they felt they knew more about my hair than I did. Then, I had other stylists that wanted to trim my hair while it was wet. I insisted that it would be better to trim my hair while dry. I told them that I preferred to have my hair trimmed while it was dry and somewhat shrunken (not wet and elongated) to ensure a more modest cut. But, no matter how much I urged them to try things differently, many of the stylists insisted on doing things their way. Some stylists even took offense at my basic suggestions. In the end, I simply thanked them for their time, passed up their services, and kept searching until I found a handful of great stylists that fit my personality and who were able to best fulfill my hair care needs.

It would be fairly accurate to say that since learning to love my hair, I have also learned to take full responsibility for my hair and avoid stylists who don't understand the importance of healthy and protective hair care. Furthermore, I've learned to not feel guilty about having a certain level of skepticism when a stylist wanted to do something that seemed a bit "off" or damaging to my hair. I've had a few nightmarish hair experiences at the hands of inexperienced stylists, and I've heard horror stories of women who experienced hair breakage, hair loss, and even scalp infections after salon visits. I've even heard stories of natural-haired women who had their hair permanently straightened by stylists who decided it would be okay to mix relaxers into deep conditioning treatments. Mind you, this was done **without the client's consent.**

When you love your hair, it's crucial that you accept responsibility for your hair. That means learning to take care of your own hair and only trusting skilled professionals with your hair care. The last thing you want to do is to put an abundance of time into growing and maintaining a healthy head of hair- only to have it damaged by someone who didn't know what they were doing.

Choosing a stylist is highly personal and very important, so use a mix of intuition and common sense. Never feel guilty about exercising a bit of caution and never be afraid to walk away from a salon or stylist if something feels off. In addition to using common sense and intuition, I would also advise you to take these factors into consideration when selecting a hair stylist.

CHOOSE STYLISTS WHO HAVE GREAT REPUTATIONS.

It's always best to use a stylist who's been referred by a trustworthy friend, family member or acquaintance. I simply don't believe in walking into random salons and seeking services from a random stylist. I feel like there's too much to chance when you do this. My hair is too precious for that, and so is yours.

CHOOSE STYLISTS WHO ARE RESPECTFUL OF YOUR TIME.

Grant it, many excellent stylists are often overbooked because everyone wants to be in their chair. Still, the sign of a professional stylist is one that will not have you waiting more than a few minutes past your appointment time. Stylists know that it's just bad business and bad manners when they overbook clients. A great stylist will always be mindful about not over-booking their appointments.

CHOOSE STYLISTS WITH CLEAN WORK STATIONS.

Hair stations and salons can get messy, especially when dealing with a large clientele. So while it's only fair to cut stylists and salons a bit of slack when it comes to work station cleanliness, it's still wise to take note of your stylist's work station and hair tools. There have been reports of individuals contracting serious bacterial scalp infections after visiting salons. And to avoid this type of issue, you want to make sure your hair is done in a work station that looks like it's been cleaned regularly.

CHOOSE STYLISTS WHO ARE GOOD LISTENERS.

A great stylist wants to keep their clients happy. Clients want to feel they are being listened to. All stylists know that a happy client means repeat business and referrals. Not wanting to listen to your needs, suggestions, or opinions, are all warning signs that a stylist may not value their relationship with you. Most importantly, these are also signs that a stylist may not even value the health of your hair.

CHOOSE STYLISTS WHO ARE GOOD COMMUNICATORS.

There's a saying that "the customer is always right." Still, there are many stylists who may know what's best for your hair. Some stylists will do whatever a client wants, while others go the extra mile to steer a client away from damaging hair practices. Either way, great stylists are those who have mastered the art of styling *and* communication. It's wonderful when you find a stylist who can work wonders with your hair, but it's even better when you find a stylist who is willing to tell you the truth about your hair, even when you may not what to hear it.

CHOOSE A STYLIST THAT YOU GENUINELY LIKE.

This may seem obvious, but I know many women that go to stylists that they don't like. I don't understand how they do it. I would never want to be stuck in a chair underneath someone that I viewed as rude, obnoxious, or antagonistic. I simply could not trust anyone like that with my hair. Furthermore, trips to the salon are a time to chill, relax and let your hair down, literally. So if you flat-out don't like your stylist or even have luke-warm feelings towards them, I'd strongly suggest that you start looking for a new stylist. It may take more time and effort, but I think it's worth it in the long run.

TAKE HOME POINTS

Take responsibility for your hair, and trust only competent stylists with your hair.

Be direct, yet respectful with stylists about your hair care needs and wants.

A great stylist will have a great reputation, be respectful of your time, be a good listener, an excellent communicator, and will have a clean work station.

A stylist should also be friendly and personable. If you do not feel completely comfortable with your current stylist, you need to find a new stylist.

CHAPTER 16
HAIR BREAKAGE & HAIR LOSS

Do you know the difference between breakage and shedding? Sometimes women confuse the two. Breakage is the result of damaged hair. Broken hair does not come out from the root. It comes from anywhere along the hair shaft that has been weakened by damage, usually the ends of the hair. As a result, breakage will appear as broken hairs of varying lengths. Shed hair, on the other hand, will be significantly longer in length. Hair sheds when it has reached the end of the growth cycle. This type of hair will fall straight from the root of the hair follicle. It will also have a hardened clear "bulb" attached near the youngest part of the hair shaft. The bulb may look white, but it is actually colorless. This bulb is called *club hair*. Club hair is what distinguishes broken hair from shed hair.

Club hair is sometimes referred to as the *hair root*. This bulb is not really the hair root. The actual hair root remains in the scalp, lodged within the hair follicle. This bulb that you see on a shed hair is part of the root sheath that has merged with the strand of hair. It is clear because it lacks melanin, the pigment that gives hair its color. The formation of club hair begins during the catagen phase of the hair growth cycle and fully forms during telogen. During this time, pigment cells will temporarily stop functioning as the hair prepares for shedding. Once this hair is shed, a new hair cycle will begin and pigment cells will start working again to help produce colored hair like before.

HAIR SHEDDING- WHAT IS NORMAL?

While hair breakage is always a sign of hair damage, hair shedding can be a normal or abnormal occurrence. In fact, it is normal to lose between 25-100 strands of hair from our heads in a given day. On the days when hair is washed, that number can go as high as 200 strands. So don't panic when you lose some hair on a daily basis. It's just the process of shedding, and in normal cases, shedding will be followed immediately by hair regrowth.

That understood, there are definitely times when you should worry about hair loss or massive hair shedding. A massive amount of hair shedding over an extended period of time, as well as a thinner appearance in your hair as time progresses, are both telltale signs that you are experiencing some form of abnormal hair loss.

Alopecia is the medical term for hair loss. There are several types of alopecia with many different causes. Some are normal causes that do not lead to permanent hair loss, such as postpartum shedding. Then there are abnormal causes of alopecia that can lead to permanent hair loss. Alopecia affects countless women of all ages and backgrounds. But, studies have shown an increased rate of certain types of alopecia in black women. This is why I felt it was important to include a chapter about it in my book.

To the average person it would seem completely ironic that black women (who make up a huge proportion of the multi-billion dollar hair industry) would also be the same women that suffer disproportionately from hair thinning and hair loss. One would logically assume that we'd have some of the thickest and healthiest hair around, especially since we're spending so much money on our hair.

The reality is that black women who rely heavily on chemical processing, heat styling and tight hair styling methods, will be at greater risk for pathological and self-induced forms of hair loss.

If you are experiencing hair thinning around your hairline, the crown of your head or on any other region of your scalp, then you may be experiencing a self-induced form of alopecia. Chemical processing, heat, and tight hairstyles are all very irritating to hair follicles. To understand why, you must realize that your hair follicles are alive. Your hair follicles are made of living cells that react to stress, internal as well as external stress. Stress in the form of chemicals, heat, and physical force, will damage hair follicles and eventually destroy them.

There are many different types of alopecia, with many different causes. I wanted to specifically address two types of alopecia that are frequently observed in black women: traction alopecia and cicatricial alopecia. Both types are typically self-induced and are very serious conditions that can lead to permanent hair loss.

TRACTION ALOPECIA

WHAT CAUSES TRACTION ALOPECIA?

Traction alopecia is caused by continuous tension on the hair for extended periods of time. This type of tension on the hair shaft will gradually cause damage to the dermal papilla and hair follicle. Traction alopecia is seen in women with natural and processed hair. It is characterized by hair thinning or hair loss around the hairline or edges, as well as above the ears. Oftentimes, women with traction alopecia will look like they have a receding hairline. This type of alopecia is commonly caused by wearing hairstyles that put tension on the hairline and hair follicles, such as ponytails, braids, buns and other hairstyles that require pulling hair back. Women who wear tight protective styles are at risk for this type of hair loss. Traction alopecia can also be caused by wearing weaves and wigs that have been secured too tightly to the hairline by glue or other strong adhesives that can literally pull the hair right out of the hair follicle when the hair piece shifts or is removed.

HOW TO PREVENT TRACTION ALOPECIA?

Women often underestimate how delicate hair is, especially the finer textured hair that exists around the hairline. Since traction alopecia is a direct result of putting stress on the hair follicle, even women who wear protective styles that put tension on the hairline will be at risk for traction alopecia.

To prevent this type of hair loss I tell women to avoid tiny and tight braids around the hairline (i.e. micro braids). I also advise women to alternate days where they wear hair pulled back and when they wear hair loose. Furthermore, when hair is pulled back the hairstyle should not be tight. For example, if you're wearing a ponytail or bun and can't take your index finger and easily loop it under the hair at your hairline, then your style is too tight and needs to be loosened.

CAN TRACTION ALOPECIA BE TREATED?

While this type of hair loss may be reversible in the **initial stages**, hair loss will be permanent if women continue unhealthy hair practices that caused the condition. Furthermore, though tension on the hair follicle is the primary cause of traction alopecia, it's also important to know that using harsh chemicals like relaxers and commercial dyes will aggravate this condition and make traction alopecia harder to treat.

CENTRAL CENTRIFUGAL CICATRICIAL ALOPECIA (CCCA)

WHAT CAUSES CENTRIFUGAL CICATRICIAL ALOPECIA?

The term centrifugal cicatricial alopecia actually refers to a diverse group of disorders that destroy the hair follicle through inflammation. These conditions are also called cicatricial alopecia for short. The exact cause of the various forms of cicatricial alopecia is not completely known. However, all forms of cicatricial alopecia do involve inflammation directed at the hair follicle. The inflammation ultimately results in destruction of the hair follicle, scar tissue formation on the scalp and permanent hair loss. Cicatricial alopecia is caused by chronic inflammation, and hair loss is sometimes accompanied by some sort of chronic itching, pain and burning of the scalp. Most often the hair thinning and hair loss will start at the crown of the head and can spread to neighboring hair follicles, resulting in an ever-enlarging area of hair loss. The hairline is usually unaffected in cases of cicatricial alopecia.

One form of cicatricial alopecia, called *hot-comb alopecia,* was first reported in the late 1960's in black women that chronically used heat styling. Cicatricial alopecia can also be seen in women who use chemical straighteners; and most chemical straighteners do contain strong agents that have the ability to burn skin, inflame the scalp and destroy hair follicles.

HOW TO PREVENT CICATRICIAL ALOPECIA?

Your scalp and hair follicles are extremely sensitive to changes in temperature and pH. Inappropriate heat styling and chemical processing will irritate and inflame the scalp, as well as the hair follicles. Heat styling and chemical processing can also alter the acid mantle, which can lead to further inflammation of the scalp through infection. Cicatricial alopecia is simply an inflammatory condition of the scalp and hair follicles. So, to reduce your risk of this type of hair loss, it would be wise to minimize or completely avoid hair practices that require frequent heat and chemical processing.

CAN CICATRICIAL ALOPECIA BE TREATED?

Being that cicatricial alopecia is a chronic inflammatory condition it is not as simple as just stopping chemical processing and heat styling. Women will have to cease all hair practices that irritate hair follicles *and* they will have to seek more advanced medical treatment. For example, women may also need to take antibiotics, prescription anti-inflammatory medications (i.e. corticosteroids), as well as other medications that have to be applied to or injected into the scalp. This is done to help alleviate follicular inflammation. As with traction alopecia, time is also of the essence when treating cicatricial alopecia. If the scalp and hair follicles are completely destroyed from inflammation before treatment, hair loss will be permanent.

TREATMENT OPTIONS FOR HAIR LOSS

There is this old saying in medicine: *an ounce of prevention is worth a pound of cure.* I think these are wise words to live by when choosing what type of hair regimen you'll follow. I've observed many women who don't want to accept that their hair practices are directly responsible for their hair issues. It's unfortunate when women live in denial about their hair practices, because in the end they just end up suffering from things like alopecia as well as other conditions that could have been easily avoided by being a bit more loving with their hair.

If you are experiencing hair loss like I've described, then it is time for you to seriously re-evaluate how you approach your hair. Your scalp and hair follicles are very delicate. You can't just abuse them and not expect a negative consequence. You must treat them with love. This is the only way to healthy hair growth. You also need to be very proactive about your hair care. If you recognize a problem with your hair or your scalp, you should be ready and willing to get to the root of the problem immediately. Ignoring the issue won't make things better. Most of the hair problems we face can be resolved, and completely avoided, if we pay attention to our hair while also maintaining a healthy and protective hair regimen.

As far as treatment options for hair loss, the results are on a case by cases basis. Not everyone will be able to re-grow their hair after it has been damaged. This is why it's best to do everything in your power to prevent hair loss from happening in the first place. Remember, *an ounce of prevention is worth a pound of cure.*

If you're experiencing hair thinning or hair loss, the best course of action is to immediately consult a dermatologist or hair specialist, such as a trichologist. Treatment options for alopecia are broken down into four main categories: cosmetic non-surgical, surgical, traditional medical, and holistic. The effects of treatment are usually based on the primary cause of hair loss and the degree of hair loss. None of these treatments have been found to be 100% effective in re-growing hair, and in all cases, treatment will require patience, time and a steadfast commitment.

COSMETIC NON-SURGICAL & SURGICAL TREATMENTS

Non-surgical treatments include wigs, weaves, scalp pencils and other methods used to *camouflage* hair loss. These treatments can be safe and effective (if used properly). Still these methods are only temporary, non-permanent solutions to hair loss. Hair transplant or hair restoration surgery, on the other hand, can be a more effective and permanent solution to hair loss. However, there are drawbacks to surgery- namely the cost. Surgical treatment can be quite expensive and it's not uncommon for patients to require multiple surgeries and many follow-up appointments before improvements in hair growth are even noticed.

TRADITIONAL & HOLISTIC MEDICAL TREATMENTS

Traditional and holistic medical treatments can be cheaper and are less invasive than surgical treatments. But once again, the results are not guaranteed. Monoxidil (brand name Rogaine) is one very popular over-the-counter FDA-approved medication that has been shown to stimulate hair growth. Minoxidil is a generic drug and is actually formulated in many other topical hair treatments besides Rogaine. Women should only use the 2% concentration of minoxidil, not the 5% formula. The FDA has not approved use of the 5% concentration for women. When using monoxidil, or any other topical hair growth treatment, patience and stead-fast commitment will be required. Results may take up to six months to show, and in the case of monoxidil, you will have to continue using this medication daily for the rest of your life. Once a person stops using monoxidil as directed, any new hair growth will gradually be lost once again.

There are also less conventional treatments for alopecia. Many of these treatments fall within the realm of alternative and holistic medicine. Alternative and holistic medicine emphasizes a more natural approach to healing. Unfortunately, both forms of medicine have not been extensively investigated by the traditional medical community. As a result, there hasn't been an abundance of evidence to prove whether they really work. Despite the lack of formal studies, there are women who have had success with stimulating hair growth by using treatments like scalp massage, aromatherapy, detoxification, nutritional supplements and herbal remedies. For example, common topical holistic treatments that have been used to stimulate hair growth include licorice, khellin, emu oil, aloe vera, grapeseed oil and Jamaican black castor oil. There are also essential oils like cedarwood, lavender, rosemary, and thyme that are infused in carrier oils like grapeseed and jojoba oil. When treating hair loss, these oils are typically massaged into the affected part of the scalp on a daily basis.

As far as nutritional supplements, they can most certainly help prevent and even reverse hair loss. Remember, healthy hair growth starts from *the inside,* and as you learned earlier, maintaining a healthy, balanced and protein-rich diet is **critical** to healthy hair growth. That understood, by supplementing your diet with high-quality nutritional supplements you can significantly improve the health and growth potential of your hair. Also, when taking a nutritional supplement you should focus on those that contain key healthy hair growth nutrients like protein, biotin, B vitamins, as well as vitamins A, C and E. You can find all of these nutrients in my advanced nutritional supplements *Beauty&Body Protein* and *Natural Beauty.* To learn more about *Beauty&Body Protein* and *Natural Beauty,* go to DRPHOENYX.COM.

Last but not least, herbal tea hair rinses are another possible treatment for hair loss. Some women swear by tea rinses and claim that they do help to prevent hair loss and stimulate hair growth. Overall herbal tea hair rinses are relatively easy to make. The tea leaves are added to hot water and then allowed steep for ten to twenty minutes. After twenty minutes, the tea is strained, cooled, and poured over freshly cleansed and conditioned hair. The tea is not rinsed from the hair. A few herbs that are frequently used for rinses include burdock, catnip, chamomile, horsetail, lavender, nettle, stinging nettle and saw palmetto. Keep in mind though that if not used carefully and as directed, certain tea rinses can expose hair follicles to an excess amount of caffeine which can stunt hair growth. So, just like any other type of holistic or alternative hair growth treatment – whether it's over the counter drugs, nutritional supplements, or tea rinses – always do your best to fully research the benefits and risks before use.

TAKE HOME POINTS

Hair breakage is not the same as hair shedding. Hair breakage is a sign of hair damage. Shed hair is a normal part of the hair growth cycle. Shed hair will have a hardened clear bulb attached near the youngest part of the hair shaft. This bulb is called club hair.

We will lose between 25-100 strands of hair from our heads in a given day. On the days when hair is washed, that number can go as high as 200 strands.

Alopecia is simply hair loss. In certain cases, alopecia can be characterized by a thinner appearance in the hair over time. There are different types of alopecia. Some types of alopecia are permanent, while others can be temporary.

Chemical processing, heat, and tight hairstyles are all very irritating to hair follicles and can cause permanent hair loss.

If you're experiencing hair thinning or hair loss, the best course of action is to immediately consult a dermatologist or trichologist. Treatment options for alopecia include: cosmetic non-surgical, surgical, medical, as well as holistic remedies like nutritional supplements.

If you'd like to learn more about hair loss and hair loss treatments, you can visit the American Hair Loss Association and the American Academy of Dermatology.

CHAPTER 17

SCALP ISSUES, DANDRUFF & DERMATITIS

Healthy hair growth can only be accomplished with a healthy scalp. This is why hair growth can become a bit problematic when you're faced with scalp issues like dandruff, itchy scalp and eczema. These conditions do have the potential to irritate your hair follicles, and as previously mentioned, an irritated scalp and irritated hair follicles can compromise hair growth. This is why it's best to immediately treat scalp conditions when they arise.

DANDRUFF

While dandruff is far from life threatening, it's still the sign of an unhealthy scalp. Dandruff indicates an imbalance in the acid mantle. Sometimes flaking from product buildup can be mistaken for dandruff, but true dandruff is due to fungal or bacterial overgrowth on the scalp and hair. The acid mantle exists to prevent the invasion and overgrowth of microorganisms on the body. In fact, your body is already home to many types of microorganisms, but the acid mantle helps to keep them in check. When the acid mantle is disturbed, balance is thrown off and certain bacteria or fungi will begin to multiply. As a result, skin will become irritated and flaky. Bacteria and fungi can even infiltrate the fibers of the hair shaft, resulting in brittle hair and breakage.

A WORD ON COMMERCIAL ANTI-DANDRUFF SHAMPOOS

Many women like to use commercial anti-dandruff shampoos. While these types of shampoos are effective at treating dandruff, they can also come with the added negative effect of significantly drying hair out. This is because many anti-dandruff shampoos contain sulfates. There are brands of highly effective dandruff shampoos that do not contain sulfates or harsh drying agents. And if you prefer using a commercial anti-dandruff shampoo you should consider checking the ingredients on the label to verify that it is sulfate-free.

NATURAL REMEDIES FOR DANDRUFF

There are many cheap, natural remedies for dandruff that are gentler and less drying than commercial products. Some of these natural remedies include aloe vera, jojoba oil and Ayurvedic herbs like neem and shika-kai. There are also essential oils like tea tree, patchouli, and rosemary that work well for treating dandruff.

If you're having issues with dandruff, you can look for commercial products that contain the herbs and oils I mentioned, or you can make your own herbal anti-dandruff treatment. Here is the recipe for a very simple and very effective anti-dandruff treatment:

HOMEMADE NEEM & TEA TREE OIL DANDRUFF TREATMENT

Mix ¼ cup of neem oil with 6 drops of tea tree oil in an applicator bottle. Apply mixture to scalp and massage. Let it sit on the hair for 10 minutes and then rinse hair. Use this treatment before cleansing hair.

DERMATITIS & ITCHY SCALP

Dermatitis means "inflammation of the skin." "Derma-" means skin and "-itis" means inflammation. The term dermatitis is very broad, and encompasses many types of skin conditions that are characterized by inflammation. Various forms of dermatitis include irritant contact dermatitis, nummular dermatitis, allergic dermatitis, seborrheic dermatitis and atopic dermatitis (i.e. eczema).

Dermatitis is classified according to the cause of the condition. Many forms of dermatitis do occur as the result of some sort of allergic reaction to a specific substance (i.e. an allergen). Although dermatitis can have many different causes, most forms of dermatitis will present with similar symptoms like swollen, reddened and itchy skin. Dermatitis can also appear anywhere on the skin, including the scalp.

On one end of the spectrum, dermatitis can be mild and simply present itself as a reddened and itchy scalp with no other major symptoms. On the other end of the spectrum, it can be a lot more bothersome and present with more aggravating symptoms- as in the case of eczema or psoriasis.

There are countless women who deal with forms of scalp dermatitis. I do empathize because years ago I suffered from a case of dermatitis and it was truly a royal pain. Fortunately, it was just a one-time flare-up, but that one-time flare-up was enough for me to make sweeping changes in my cosmetic products. I haven't had an issue with my skin since.

As stated earlier, dermatitis can be due to some type of allergen exposure. This allergen could be a harsh chemical in a cosmetic product, body soap or even laundry detergent. The allergic response could also be the result of exposure to dust mites or even pet dander. In most cases, dermatitis will not be a serious medical condition. But when located on the scalp, this inflammatory condition can lead to hair loss as a result of follicular inflammation and scar formation due to chronic scratching.

When treating dermatitis, I recommend three courses of action:

1. Consider using more natural or hypoallergenic hair care and skin products.

2. Consider using hypoallergenic household detergents (i.e. soaps and laundry detergent).

3. Consider modifying your diet.

Oftentimes chemicals, dyes and perfumes in commercial products can be very aggravating to certain skin types. Studies have shown that preservatives, artificial dyes, and other chemicals in cosmetic products can cause dermatitis. For this reason, if you are suffering from chronic dermatitis it may be wise to consider switching to more natural or organic hair care products. You may also want to refrain from chemically processing your hair. If you are having issues with dermatitis, but still want to use commercial products, I'd suggest that you only use hypoallergenic products. A product will be labeled as hypoallergenic if it is formulated without harsh chemicals and ingredients that can irritate the skin.

After opting for more natural and hypoallergenic products, I'd also suggest regularly washing all clothes and linens with a hypoallergenic brand of laundry detergent. You should also invest in a water filter or water softener since hard water can irritate skin.

There are many natural remedies for dermatitis and generally itchy scalp. A few topical remedies that may help to further soothe irritation include neem, bhringraj, brahmi, marshmallow root, tea tree oil, lavender oil, chamomile, peppermint oil, jojoba oil, emu oil, and evening primrose oil. In addition to topical treatments there are also dietary modifications and nutritional supplements that may help with dermatitis. Remember, your skin is a reflection of your health. So, it may be wise to consider modifying your diet in favor of more whole foods, less processed foods, less dairy foods, and more gluten-free foods (gluten allergy has been linked to cases of eczema and other forms of dermatitis).

As far as supplements, omega fatty acids are frequently used to promote healthy skin and a healthy scalp. Regularly taking an omega-3 supplement like fish oil may also help to improve symptoms of dermatitis.

I would recommend that you try any of these recommendations for a few weeks and see how they work. It may take some time to get to the root cause of dermatitis so be patient. If you still don't see improvement in your condition after 6-8 weeks, it would be wise to also seek medical treatment from your doctor.

TAKE HOME POINTS

Healthy hair growth first requires a healthy scalp.

Dandruff is a sign of fungal overgrowth on the scalp and hair. Natural remedies for dandruff include aloe vera, jojoba oil, tea tree oil and neem.

If you use a commercial anti-dandruff shampoo, make sure it is sulfate-free.

Dermatitis means inflammation of the skin. There are many different forms of dermatitis with variable forms of treatment.

Many forms of dermatitis are due to allergen exposure. Allergens can be harsh chemicals, preservatives, and artificial dyes found in cosmetics, soaps and detergents.

When treating dermatitis, you should consider using more natural or hypoallergenic products and modifying your diet.

CHAPTER 18

WEAVES, WIGS AND HAIR EXTENSIONS

There's no denying that weaves, wigs and extensions can be great for protective styling while letting you maintain an incredibly fabulous look. But, they do have their dark side. If worn incorrectly these hair accessories can cause serious scalp issues, hair breakage, alopecia, and worst yet, make you look a hot mess.

Weaves, wigs and hair extensions are not something to drop on your head without much forethought, care, or precaution. A lot can go wrong if you do. Prolonged pulling at hair strands from tight or heavy hairpieces can cause hair breakage and hair loss. If going bald isn't bad enough, women also add insult to injury when they rock hair pieces that *also* end up looking a hot mess from poor maintenance and poor hair hygiene. We've all seen those ratty, bird's nest-looking weaves and wigs. Not a good look!

When wearing hairpieces, you have to pay very close attention to *your* hair, as well as the styling and maintenance of your *other* hair. To make things less confusing, let's call your other hair *Sasha*.

When wearing a hairpiece, you have to strike a balance where your hair and Sasha can coexist in perfect harmony. Here are a few suggestions on how to do this:

CHOOSE HUMAN HAIR

Sasha will most likely come in both synthetic and natural hair types. Synthetic hair (i.e. plastic hair) is a common, cheaper choice, but it may irritate your skin and lead to an allergic reaction. I once had a lady ask me why her forehead, neck and scalp were breaking out in itchy bumps. She'd never experienced anything like it before. After a few more questions, it was revealed that she had recently purchased a wig made with synthetic hair. The synthetic wig looked great, but it ended up causing an allergic skin reaction. In the end, this woman ended up having to see a doctor for treatment. This is a very common example of why it's probably best to buy Sasha in human hair. It may be a bit more expensive, but your skin and hair are worth it.

WATCH YOUR HAIRLINE, LOOSEN UP AND BE MINDFUL OF HEAVY EXTENSIONS

Here's a bit of advice on wearing hairpieces: Never use glue to hold Sasha in place. And never, ever, ever wear Sasha so tight that you need to take an aspirin while she's on. These are some of the quickest ways to thin your hairline and cause permanent hair loss. In addition, if Sasha comes in the form of braids or any type of hair extension, you want to be very careful about the amount of hair that you add to your actual hair. Your hair strands are anchored into the hair follicle. Braids and hair extensions cause alopecia because they break this anchor between the hair strand and the hair follicle. Hair follicles are designed to only withstand a certain amount of force and tension at the hair root. As the weight of your hair increases from heavy hair extensions, the tension on the root of your hair will also increase. With enough tension, your hair's anchor will give way.

There are many women who like to wear extensions to create a fuller look. Unfortunately, they may end up making themselves bald in the process. If you don't want this to happen to you as well, make sure to watch your hairline, loosen up, and ease up on the amount of hair. Sasha is cool and all, but enough times of wearing her incorrectly, and you may end up *needing* to wear Sasha more than you'd like.

DON'T NEGLECT YOUR HAIR

You can't just slap Sasha on your head and forget about your own hair. You will still need to regularly cleanse and condition your hair, as well as your scalp. If you don't do this, your hair will become dry, brittle and break. Furthermore, it's not healthy or hygienic to allow buildup of oil, dirt, hair products and bacteria on your scalp. Wearing weaves, wigs and hair accessories can create a dark, moist environment on the scalp that can become a breeding ground for bacteria and fungus. The overgrowth of these types of microorganisms can lead to smelly hair, dandruff, serious scalp infections, and even hair loss.

UPGRADE YOUR HAIR PRODUCTS

Truth be told, even if you aren't wearing Sasha, you should already use the best products you can find for your hair and scalp. Upgrading your hair products doesn't mean that you have to switch to only expensive, brand name products. Upgrading just means that you need to pay close attention to product ingredients. Now is the time to avoid products with ingredients like sodium lauryl sulfate, alcohol, and synthetic emollients. In addition, you should look towards using more natural products, like tea tree oil and lavender oil, which promote healthy hair growth and also have antiseptic properties that guard against fungal and bacterial overgrowth.

DON'T SLACK OFF ON YOUR HEALTH

Sasha should never be an excuse for you to skip the gym or slack off on your eating habits. Sometimes she does provide a bit of an escape from the work that goes into growing and caring for hair on a daily basis, but always remember that proper nutrition and exercise are cornerstones to hair growth. Healthy hair starts from the inside out. So when wearing

Sasha, don't forget to continue nourishing your body and *your* hair with a healthy diet and healthy lifestyle. Remember, Sasha has to come off at some point, and you still want your natural hair to be there, healthy and strong, when she does.

KNOW WHEN TO BREAK UP WITH SASHA

It may be a hard thing to accept, but sometimes Sasha isn't the best girlfriend to have. Sometimes she can end up damaging your hair. There was a time when Sasha helped you look fierce, but now she's also causing breakage, hair thinning and hair loss. When this happens, it will be time to put Sasha aside and tell her that you two need to take a break. It doesn't have to be a permanent break-up per se. But, I'd recommend that you take a relationship break for at least six months until you can resolve your hair and/or scalp issues. Be strong enough to walk away from Sasha if she's damaging your hair. In time, you may be able to eventually reconcile with Sasha, however I would only do so after you've completely resolved all of your hair growth issues.

Overall, I think this is where many women go wrong with hair care in general. They notice a deterioration in the health of their hair, but keep doing the same things that caused their hair problems. Don't make the same mistake. If you notice that Sasha is damaging your hair, don't be afraid to break up with her. You can love Sasha all you like, but you still need to love your hai more.

TAKE HOME POINTS

Improperly worn weaves, wigs and hair extensions can cause serious scalp infections and hair loss.

When using weaves, wigs and hair extensions you should be mindful about the type of hair you use, how tightly the hair is secured into place, how often you cleanse and condition your hair, and the types of hair products that you use.

Maintain a healthy diet and a healthy haircare regimen, like regularly cleansing your hair and scalp, even when wearing weaves and wigs.

Consult a doctor and immediately cease using any weave, wig or hair extension if you notice any type of scalp infection, scalp inflammation and/or hair loss.

CHAPTER 19

FOR THE NEW NATURAL

For the newly natural women who are reading this book, I just have one thing to say: Congrats! Going natural is truly an awesome experience. Writing this book brought back so many memories of my natural hair journey. As I wrote the chapters, particularly *My Hair Story*, I vividly recalled how empowering and challenging it was, especially for a woman like myself. I had worn a relaxer most of my life. It had been this way for so long that my relaxed hair had become "normal" and my afro-textured hair had become "foreign." I knew nothing about caring for my natural hair. There was so much new information to take in. Ultimately, I did come to a point in my life where I learned to love and care for my natural hair. The whole experience was so transforming, and writing about it in this book has been a wonderful trip down memory lane.

When I went natural, it wasn't as popular as it is now. Today, it seems like every day I'm meeting women who are making the transition to natural hair. And I think it's awesome! So in celebration of this, I decided to include a chapter specifically for the newly natural, *as well* as those who are contemplating taking the natural plunge. I'll just review the ways you can go natural, offer a few additional hair care tips, and also offer suggestions on what you need *before* going natural. Now let's first take a closer look at how women can go from relaxed to natural hair.

GOING NATURAL- TRANSITION & BIG CHOP

There are two ways to go natural: transition or big chop. Transitioning involves growing your hair out, while gradually trimming your relaxed ends. After enough trims, you will reach a point where there's no longer any relaxed hair left to cut. The concept of transitioning is pretty straight-forward. Just trim your hair at your own discretion. The duration or length of the entire transitioning process is totally up to you.

The other option to going natural is known as the "big chop." This is exactly what it sounds like. You cut off all of your relaxed hair in one clean swoop. The big chop can result in a short fade or a teeny-weeny afro, depending on whether you already started growing out your relaxer beforehand.

There are pros and cons to transitioning and the big chop. Most women choose based on their personality and hair preferences. The big chop is often seen as a more drastic option, especially for women who may be used to longer hair. Still, many women love the big chop experience and find it to be more liberating because it allows them to jump right into natural hair. However, the big chop may come with certain frustrations. While many women love their new shorter 'dos, I have also heard women complain that they feel less feminine with short hair. Then, there are issues with limited styling options. Still, I think it's all a matter of perception and willingness to work with what you've got.

The big chop is a great time to embrace your inner diva and play up your other physical features by wearing makeup and even rocking cute earrings and jewelry. Hair isn't the only beautiful feature you have. You have your eyes, your lips, your cheekbones and your entire physique for that matter. Furthermore, having shorter hair will allow you to start appreciating and showcasing other features that may have been overlooked before. Overall, the big chop can be a very bold move in itself and can push women to develop a stronger sense of self-awareness and self-confidence.

Transitioning is a more gradual process for women who'd rather "ease into" natural hair. Some women want to go natural, but they don't want to sacrifice length. I can certainly understand and respect this perspective; however, transitioning does come with unique challenges. When transitioning, you will be dealing with two types of hair, relaxed and natural. So a big issue with transitioning hair is breakage. This happens because the demarcation point between natural and relaxed hair is very weak. This weakness is the result of a lack of uniformity in the cortical structure. Remember, relaxers change the structure of cortex. So when growing out a relaxer, you will have a strand of hair with two different cortical structures- one weaker than the other. And oftentimes, when transitioning hair is manipulated, it will break. Styling is another challenge with transitioning hair because there will be one part of the hair that's straight and another part that's curly or kinky

The best way to work around transition issues of breakage and styling is to be extremely mindful of regularly moisturizing and deep conditioning. You want to moisturize daily and deep condition at least once a week. Conditioner, leave-in conditioner and moisturizer should become your BFF during the transition process. This type of regimen will help to reinforce the strength and elasticity of hair through protein-moisture balancing. Breakage will always be an issue with transitioning hair, but the more you can help to keep your hair strong and elastic, the longer you will be able to grow it out before breakage becomes extensive. As far as styling options, hair that's in transition is best worn in curlier styles that will help to blend your two types of hair. Perm rod sets, roller sets, braid-outs, twist-outs, braids, and kinky twists are all easy ways to blend two types of hair. If you are looking for more styling options, check out videos on YouTube. There are many wonderful natural hair vloggers who offer tips for styling transitioning hair.

One thing women should not do when transitioning is use heat styling as a way to blend their two hair types. I have seen many women transition to natural hair while using things like flat irons to blend their two textures of hair. This is one of the worst things you can do and is completely counterproductive to healthy hair growth. When transitioning, you should completely avoid heat styling. Remember, the damage that occurs from heat styling is irreversible, which means you'll irreversibly damage your new growth. Furthermore, when you regularly heat style you will be more likely to reach your *critical length* before you reach your hair's *maximum growth potential*. This is why it is best to go for curlier styles and conform to your natural hair's curl and texture when transitioning. Don't try to conform to your straighter, relaxed hair because this hair will eventually be trimmed away.

Both methods of going natural come with their own benefits and drawbacks. You just have to be flexible and embrace the ups and downs that come with each. Furthermore, it's not set in stone that you have to continue on one path or another. For example, there are women who start out transitioning, but ultimately end up doing a big chop because they grew frustrated with breakage and dealing with two different types of hair. There are also those women who go for the big chop, and then start wearing weaves or wigs because they want longer styles from time to time. All and all, this is a highly personal and very flexible process.

Before moving on in this chapter I also want to emphasize another important point. After my big chop, I quickly learned that natural hair does not automatically lead to the hair goals I sought after. Yes, my new natural hair was, in the general sense, stronger than my previously processed hair. But it took more than simply having natural hair to achieve my hair goals. What will ultimately determine your ability to achieve longer and healthier hair is how loving and protective you are with your hair. This is why I follow a protective hair regimen and I also practice lifestyle principles, like maintaining a healthy diet for healthy hair growth. And if you too are serious about your hair goals, I would strongly encourage you to be mindful about how you approach your hair. If you don't follow a protective regimen and have sound lifestyle principles, it will be harder to achieve maximum health and growth potential with your hair.

A WORD ON SHRINKAGE, TANGLING & STRETCHING

All newly natural women will notice a considerable difference in the length of their hair when it's wet versus when it's dry. Welcome to the wonderful world of shrinkage! It's not uncommon to take a strand of curly hair that's shoulder length, stretch it, and then realize that it's true length reaches almost mid-back!

Some women love their natural hair but really dislike shrinkage because it makes it harder for them to enjoy and show-off their hard-earned length. If you have natural hair, you just have to accept that shrinkage comes with the territory. There are ways to counteract shrinkage, but before I get to that I wanted to address one major issue that could arise with shrinkage- tangling. When hair shrinks and bunches up on itself, tangling could become an issue. So aside from making hair look shorter than it really is, shrinkage can make natural hair maintenance a bit more challenging due to tangling.

When I had straightened hair, tangling was not a frequent occurrence or much of a hair issue. I still had many other hair issues, but I must admit that tangling was not one of them. Many women who cross over to natural hair will be so used to working with straightened hair that it can become overwhelming and even exhausting when they have to detangle and style their curlier, coiler and kinkier natural hair. Years of caring for straightened hair may leave some women lacking the skills *and* **patience** needed to care for a different type of hair.

One of the inescapable characteristics of curly and kinky hair is that it will tangle more easily than straight hair. This does not mean it is in any way "inferior" to straight hair. It just means that curly and kinky hair is different and needs to be approached differently for styling and maintenance.

As far as methods to reduce shrinkage and tangling, there are a few. Banding is a technique used to "stretch" natural hair and elongate the curl pattern. In addition to banding, other options for stretching natural hair include threading (also known as the Ghana plait technique), as well as twisting, braiding, roller-setting hair and "pineappling." All of these stretching methods are used to prevent shrinkage by temporarily elongating the hair strand and creating a fuller or bigger looking Afro or hairstyle.

With the exception of pineappling, you should make sure to wet the hair first if you choose to stretch your hair by any of the above methods. Wet setting hair will help to elongate the hair shaft as much as possible. As far as wetting methods, hair can be washed and conditioned or dampened with a leave-in conditioner. Also make sure to give hair enough time to fully dry. Depending on how thick or long your hair is, it may take several hours for hair to fully dry and set into its stretched state. One key thing to note about banding, threading, twists and braids is that they will also leave their own distinctive and temporary pattern in the hair when taken out. This is something to keep in mind if you are trying to achieve a particular style.

Stretching hair is all personal preference and it is not a necessity. Furthermore, having shrinkage doesn't necessarily mean you'll always have an issue with tangling. Some women like to stretch their hair and some women don't. Personally, I am not a fan of any type of stretching method that requires putting tension on the roots of the hair or tight-fitting accessories on the hair shaft itself. So if you decide to stretch your hair in this type of manner I would say to be careful and do it sparingly. While this type of stretching method may work, it can also greatly increase the risk of hair damage and possible hair loss.

A WORD ON DAILY WASH-AND-GO

One of the best things about having natural hair is being able to literally jump in the shower, wash your hair, and go! Women, especially those that previously wore relaxers, often rave about the newfound freedom that they feel with natural hair. One of my biggest joys when going natural was no longer having the ever-burdening fear of getting my hair wet. It's so nice to jump in the shower every day and wet my hair without a care in the world.

There are many natural haired women who really enjoy washing their hair every morning, but I don't like to wash my hair on a daily basis for a few important reasons.

Before I get to those reasons I wanted to address a common misconception that washing hair frequently dries it out. Assuming that you're not dealing with an issue of hard water, frequently washing your hair will not dry it out. To the contrary, frequently washing hair could be a good thing because water will work as a source of constant moisture. The issue with washing hair frequently typically comes with the products you're using. If you're using products with harsh ingredients, then frequently washing your hair will most certainly be a bad thing.

Even though I use pretty good hair products and a water filter, I still avoid frequent washing. I do this because I believe it can be the enemy to growth due to constant tinkering with hair's acid mantle and protein-moisture balance. Furthermore, frequent manipulation through cleansing and styling will also accelerate the rate of hair damage. When you wash-and-go on a daily basis, you frequently expose your hair to the 3H's, especially hygral fatigue. Even if you pre-poo, this doesn't guarantee your hair will be 100% protected. Pre-poo is not an impenetrable armor on your hair shaft, and it still requires that you manipulate your hair. Remember, more manipulation equals more opportunity for damage. Thus washing your hair on a daily basis may not be a good idea if you're looking to gain maximum length with your hair. As nice as wash-and-go can be, it is possible to overdue a good thing.

6 THINGS YOU'LL NEED BEFORE GOING NATURAL

As exciting and alluring as it can be, I will stress that going natural is not something you should do on a whim, especially if you've never cared for natural hair before. You'll first need to thoroughly think it through while anticipating certain challenges that may arise. Natural hair does not behave like relaxed hair. So, before going natural, I strongly advise that you start educating yourself about natural hair care. Talk to natural-haired women about what they do for their hair. Take your time to learn as much as you can about the whole process. Whenever someone gives you advice, write it down so you can refer to it later. As a woman with natural hair, I will tell you that the road to natural is wonderful, but it is also paved with occasional obstacles. If you're seriously interested in going natural, the best thing you can do is start preparing yourself for the experience now. In the meantime, I'll also share six things that you'll need *before* going natural.

1. LOVE FOR YOUR OWN HAIR & REALISTIC EXPECTATIONS.

Before going natural, many women will look at another natural woman's hair and immediate declare, *"I want that!"* They'll get pumped up, start transitioning, or go for the big chop, and expect their hair to grow in *exactly* like their hair idol. Unfortunately, there can be great deal of disappointment when this newly natural woman discovers that her hair doesn't seem to want to look quite like someone else's. This is why I always emphasize loving *your* hair. Always come from a place of love and acceptance with your hair. Coming from a place of love will help you to have more realistic expectations about your hair. Remember, each head of hair is unique, and going natural should be about you looking like *YOU*- not you looking like someone else.

A Word on Hair Envy

Hair envy is something that can become destructive in your natural hair journey. While it's fine to admire another woman's hair, you shouldn't come from a place of envy. When you come from a place of envy, you'll never feel fulfilled. You shouldn't feel the need to look like another woman in order to feel beautiful.

Let me use myself as an example. I love Tanika Ray's hair. She's been one of my hair idols for many years, but even with all the admiration I have for Tanika Ray's hair, I can still recognize that I will never have her hair, and I'm fine with that. Furthermore, I do not view my hair as inferior to her hair, or anyone else's hair for that matter. I truly love my hair. And other women with gorgeous hair simply serve as an example of how diverse and beautiful hair can be.

My overall point is that hair envy is not healthy. It is rooted in insecurity and it can be destructive. It puts you in a place where you'll view your hair as inferior. Constantly comparing your hair to others just leads down a road to ultimately believing that your hair is less than. But, you and your hair are never less than. Furthermore, we women need to remember that beauty is not solely defined by our exterior. Skin will eventually wrinkle and the luster of hair will fade, but it is our inner beauty that never escapes us. So, while it's okay to admire what others have, always cherish and love what YOU have above anything else.

2. CONFIDENCE & ENCOURAGEMENT

When going natural, you will need confidence and encouragement. It's not uncommon for newly natural women to face negative and insulting remarks from friends and even family members. When I went natural, I experienced negative comments from a handful of people very close to me. This kind of negativity can be very discouraging and even depressing. Unfortunately, there are people in the world that, for whatever reason, don't like natural hair. I've read and heard many stories of women and young girls who've had to suffer through the negativity of people who not only disliked natural hair, but also felt the need to discourage others from wearing their hair in its natural state. This is a very hot-button topic within the black and Latino community. That stated, I wanted to offer my sincere opinion on the topic and share a bit of advice.

We live in a society flooded with images of a certain "standard of beauty." Whether it's lighter skin or straighter hair, overall the standard sends a clear and persistent message of what is perceived by society to be most attractive. The message is internalized subconsciously and the effects are played out in every day conversations. Think of how many times you've heard a person of color say "she has good hair" when referring to a woman with curly or "multi-racial"-looking hair. While this comment may seem completely innocent or nonchalant, what kind of message does a comment like this send to a little girl or woman who does not have the same type and texture of hair as the woman with "good hair?"

Without a doubt, there are people all around us who have been conditioned to believe that their natural beauty is not worthy of acknowledgment and praise. Some people of color have come to idolize the standard of beauty so much so that they consciously and subconsciously curse the very skin, hair and body they've been blessed with. But, it doesn't stop there. Sometimes the very same people who feel unworthy and unattractive may even try to spread their feelings of inferiority by belittling their own race or culture. It's a disturbing behavior that many of us have observed. For example, it's amazing how many times I've encountered a black person who has tried to put down a black woman for wearing her hair in its natural state.

Will all people of color ever come to a point where we're totally accepting of our natural beauty? I honestly don't know the answer to that question. Furthermore, the greater reality of the situation is that people all over the world suffer from inferiority complexes. It's really a universal problem that crosses cultural, race and gender lines.

This is why we women, young and old, regardless of race or culture need to accept ourselves and be who we want to be regardless of what other people may think or idolize.

Love yourself and be your biggest cheerleader in life. In life there will be people who don't like how you look. Those people may even look *just like you*. Don't concern yourself with them, their issues or dislikes. Don't let ignorance or fear stop you from being who you want to be. In the end, negativity is just noise and nonsense. It's like bad frequency on a radio, so just change the station and tune it out.

I often think back to my girlfriend in high school and how see proudly and unapologetically wore hear natural hair despite what others had to say. At such a young age she displayed grace and confidence that we should all aspire to. Think of it this way ladies: Is it really worth limiting your happiness because *you've chosen* to stress yourself out over what other people think of you?

Along with maintaining a strong sense of self-confidence, one of the best things you can do to help you along in your natural hair journey is to look towards other natural-haired women for inspiration and encouragement. Put up pictures of natural-haired women. Set personal hair goals, document your hair journey with photos and even consider writing about your experience in a journal. You should also talk to women who understand what you're going through. Make friends with other natural-haired women. Start a natural hair group, join a natural hair group, and participate in online forums. There are natural-haired women everywhere who share similar hair experiences, and many are eager to support, teach, and learn from one another. Regardless of what anyone has to say, this is the hair you've been blessed with. It's beautiful just the way it is and don't ever feel like you can't wear your hair the way it naturally grows out of your head.

3. OPEN-MINDEDNESS

I just touched on inferiority complexes and how others may try to discourage you from embracing your natural hair. Now, I want to touch on how some women with natural hair may become a bit insensitive towards women who choose to relax their hair.

While it's one thing to share information about natural hair, I think it's important to maintain a sense of humility about your and everyone else's hair choices. As much as you should love and celebrate your natural hair, I also think it's important to refrain from becoming judgmental. You can be proud of your natural hair and share information about natural hair care while also maintaining a sense of open-mindedness about everyone else's hair choices. At the end of the day, every woman should have the freedom to express her beauty the way she deems fit, whether it's via an Afro or relaxed hair. It's hard enough learning to love and accept ourselves despite the criticism and judgment of others. And we women should strive to encourage and celebrate each other, regardless of how we wear our hair.

4. HELP FINDING A STYLIST

I offered suggestions on how to select a hair stylist, and I'll also add that when going natural you will absolutely need to use a stylist that is specifically trained in caring for natural hair. Don't trust just any stylist with your hair, and absolutely avoid stylists who seem unsure of themselves or who flat out tell you that they don't know how to care for natural hair.

Depending on where you live, it may be a bit difficult to find a great natural hair stylist. This is why I'd suggest looking for a natural hair stylist now, before you go natural. You may not know of any stylists that specialize in natural hair, and this is where your natural support system is going to come into play. Start asking other natural-haired women for stylist and salon referrals. Asking for referrals now will make things a lot easier if you need to seek professional services later.

5. PATIENCE

Going natural requires lots of patience. Many women report a period in their natural hair journey when they felt incredibly frustrated and even contemplated going back to relaxers because they didn't immediately achieve the results they wanted. If you ever get this feeling, rest assured, you're not alone. It's just a rough patch.

If you truly want to go the natural route you need to understand that this process will take time and patience. But, if length is something you desperately crave, then I recommend protective styling with extensions, or even a weave, while allowing your natural hair to grow in. After a few weeks, you should remove your weave and take a few days to play in your hair. Have fun with your new curls, coils and kinks. Enjoy your natural hair and celebrate all the freedom that comes with it.

6. WILLINGNESS TO LEARN- A LOT!

Going natural requires learning a lot of the things you may have never known about hair. Your hair will not behave like it did when it was relaxed, so start checking out online forums like Facebook, YouTube, Twitter, Tumblr, Fotki, and also feel free to hit me up if you have any questions. There's a ton of information out there. You just need to be proactive, excited about this process and eager to learn. It's this enthusiasm and diligence that will carry you along on the great and not-so-great hair days. Embrace the journey, get excited about it and take in all the knowledge you can. This will make your natural hair experience a lot less complicated, and a lot more fun!

TAKE HOME POINTS

There are two ways to go natural: transition or big chop. Transitioning involves growing your hair out, while gradually trimming your relaxed ends. The big chop involves cutting off all relaxed or processed hair in one sitting.

Transitioning to natural hair does come with unique challenges because you will be dealing with two types of hair, relaxed and natural. The two biggest challenges with transitioning hair are breakage and styling options.

When transitioning you want to be extremely mindful of regularly moisturizing and deep conditioning. You want to regularly use conditioner, leave-in conditioner and moisturizer to reinforce the hair and off-set breakage.

When transitioning, it is best to wear hair in curlier styles that will help to blend your two types of hair. Perm rod sets, roller sets, braid-outs, twist-outs, braids, and kinky twists are all easy ways to blend two types of hair. Do not use heat styling as a way to blend your two hair types.

When stretching hair, be very careful and mindful of the technique used. While a particular stretching method may work, it could also greatly increase the risk of hair damage and possible hair loss.

Wash-and-go on a daily basis will accelerate hair damage and increase the risk of breakage. It is best to not wash hair too frequently, especially when transitioning to natural hair.

Going natural is an exciting process and it is also something you should prepare for. There will be emotional and physical challenges. So thoroughly think the process through *before* committing and start educating yourself about natural hair care today.

CHAPTER 20
FINAL THOUGHTS

Well ladies, we've finally reached the end! But, this really isn't the end per se. It's just the beginning of your individual hair journeys. I hope you enjoyed this book and found the information within both helpful and inspiring.

Women frequently ask me questions about hair, so I used these inquiries as inspiration for writing this book. When I first sat down to write this book, I knew that I wanted to give women something that was informative, while also giving a glimpse into my own personal hair story. In some ways, I even wrote this book as if I was writing it for *myself* or more specifically, my younger self many years ago when I had so many questions about healthy hair growth.

A lot of love went into this book and I truly enjoyed the experience. I've been a writer for many years, and I knew writing was my passion after penning my first short story in the fifth grade. The story was for a writing contest, and I actually have the award certificate I won for that very same contest framed above the fireplace in my home. It serves as an homage to that little girl who said *"one day, I'm going to be an author!"* This book is the physical manifestation of a lifelong dream, and the first book of more to come! This is something that came from my heart, and I thank you immensely for taking the time to read my hair story and my book. I'd love your feedback so please leave reviews about my book on Amazon, Barnes and Noble, or wherever you purchased it. Even if you stole the book from your girlfriend, still leave a review. I'd love to know what you all thought about my book! If you'd like to keep up with me and get a regular dose of fitness, natural beauty and healthy living tips, be sure to check out my blog and my YouTube channel. Last but not least, go to my website, DRPHOENYX.COM, to order my nutritional supplements for healthy hair growth, and be sure to also check out my supercute children's book, *Love Your Hair*!

In closing, I wish you all the best on your healthy hair and your health living journeys. Remember, healthy and longer hair is always in your reach. It just takes time, patience and commitment. If you love it, it will grow!

REFERENCES

HAIR GROWTH

Dermatologic Therapy. (2004). (Volume 17, Number 2, J pp. 164-176)

Frangie, Catherine M. (2008). *Milady's Standard Cosmetology*. USA: Thompson Delmar Learning.

Gray, John (1997). *The World of Hair: A Scientific Companion*. New York: Delmar.

Halal, John (2002). *Hair Structure and Chemistry Simplified, 4th Ed.* USA: Milady

Leading Causes of Death in Females – United States. (2007). *Centers for Disease Control and Prevention.* Retrieved from http://www.cdc.gov/women/lcod.

Marian Wright Edelman to Speak at Meharry Medical College Commencement. (2008). *Nashville Business Journal.*

Paus, Ralf. (1999). *The Biology of Hair Follicles.* The New England Journal of Medicine. 341(7).

Quadflieg, Jutta Maria. (2003). Fundamental Properties of Afro-American Hair as Related to Their Straightening/Relaxing Behaviour. Retrieved from http://sylvester.bth.rwth-aachen.de/dissertationen/2004/094/04_094.pdf

Stenn, K.S. & Paus, Ralf. (2001). Controls of Hair Follicle Cycling. Physiological Reviews 81 (1): 449-494.

Walker, Andre. (1997). *Andre Walker Talks Hair.* New York: Simon & Schuster

HAIR DAMAGE

Brown, V., Crounse, R., Abele, D. (1986). An unusual new hair shaft abnormality: "bubble hair". *Journal of American Academy of Dermatology*.

Detwiler S. P., Carson J. L., Woolsey J. T., et al. (1994). *Bubble hair: Case caused by an overheating hair dryer and reproducibility in normal hair with heat.* Journal of American Academy of Dermatology.

Elston, D. M., Bergfeld, W. F., Whiting, D. A., Mcmahon, J. T., Dawson, D. M., Quint, K. L., & Muhlbauer, J. E. (1992). Bubble hair. *Journal of Cutaneous Pathology*, doi:10.1111/1600-0560. ep11850544

Gummer C. (1994). *Bubble hair: a cosmetic abnormality caused by brief, focal heating of damp hair fibres.* British Journal of Dermatology.

US Geological Survey. Retrieved from http://www.usgs.gov/

NUTRITION

Alternative Medicine Review. (2003). *Methylsulfonylmethane (MSM).* Thorne Research, Inc. Institute of Medicine (IOM). Dietary Reference Intakes: Tolerable Upper Intake Levels. *The National Academies Press.* Retrieved from http://www. iom.edu/Activities/Nutrition/SummaryDRIs/~/media/Files/Activity%20 Files/Nutrition/DRIs/ULs%20for%20Vitamins%20and%20Elements. pdf

Institute of Medicine (IOM). (2005). "Source of Acceptable Macronutrient Distribution Range (AMDR) Reference and RDAs," in Dietary Reference Intakes for Energy, Carbohydrate, Fiber, Fat, Fatty Acids, Cholesterol, Protein and Amino Acids. *The National Academies Press.* Retrieved from http://www.iom.edu/Global/News%20Announcements/~/media/ C5CD2DD7840544979A549EC47E56A02B.ashx

Jackson, Sheila. (1985). *Anatomy & Physiology for Nurses.* Nurses' Aids Series (9th ed.). London: Bailliere Tindall.

Lawrence, Ronald M, M.D, Pd.D. (2004). Clinical Trial Report: The Effectiveness of the Use of Oral Lignisul MSM (Methylsulfonylmethane) Supplementation on Hair and Nail Health. *Carolwood Corporation.* Retrieved from http://www.essential-foods.co.uk/MSM-Studien/Lawrence-Hair-Nail-Report.htm

Office of Dietary Supplements. (2011). Dietary Supplements: What You Need to Know. *National Institutes of Health.* Retrieved from http://ods.od.nih.gov/

Tufts Medical Center. (2011). Methyl Sulfonyl Methane (MSM). Retrieved from http://www.tuftsmedicalcenter.org/apps/Healthgate/Article.aspx?chunkiid=21691

University of Maryland Medical Center. (2009). *Vitamins: An Introduction.* Retrieved from http://www.umm.edu/patiented/articles/what_vitamins_000039_1.htm

Weil, Andrew M.D. Gamma-Linolenic Acid. *DrWeil.com.* Retrieved from http://www.drweil.com/drw/u/id/ART00363

Weil, Andrew M.D. Six Tips for Healthy Hair and Skin. *DrWeil.com.* Retrieved from http://www.drweil.com/drw/u/ART02032/healthy-hair-and-skin.html

Zelman, Kathleen. The Wonders of Water. *WebMD.* Retrieved from http://www.webmd.com/diet/guide/wonders-of-water

BREAKING DOWN HAIR PRODUCTS

Davies, S. J. J. F. (1963). "Emus". *Australian Natural History.* 14: 225–229.

Frangie, Catherine M. (2008). Milady's Standard Cosmetology. USA: Thompson Delmar Learning.

NATURAL EMOLLIENTS

Cooksley, V. G. (1996). *Aromatherapy: A Lifetime Guide to Healing with Essential Oils.* New Jersey: Prentice Hall Press.

Emerit I, Filipe P, Freitas J, Vassy J. (2004). Protective effect of superoxide dismutase against hair graying in a mouse model. *Photochemistry and photobiology.* 80:579–582. Retrieved from http://www.ncbi.nlm.nih.gov/pubmed/15623346

Inoue, T., Ito, M., & Kizawa, K. (2002). Labile proteins accumulated in damaged hair upon permanent waving and bleaching treatments. Journal of Cosmetic Science. Retrieved from http://journal.scconline.org/pdf/cc2002/cc053n06/p00337-p00344.pdf

Journal of Cosmetic Science. (2001). "Penetrating vs. Non-penetrating Oils." (pp. 169-84)

Keville, Kathi. (1998). *Herbs for Health and Healing.* New York: Berkley Books.

Rele & Mohile. (2002). Effect of mineral oil, sunflower oil, and coconut oil on prevention of hair damage. *Journal of Cosmetic Science.* Retrieved from http://journal.scconline.org/pdf/cc2003/ cc054n02/p00175-p00192.pdf

Ruetsch, S. B., Kamath, Y. K., Rele, A. S., & Mohile, R. B. (2001). Secondary Ion Mass Spectrometric Investigation of Penetration of Coconut and Mineral Oils into Human Hair Fibers: Relevance to Hair Damage. *Journal of Cosmetic Science.*

Wertz, P.W. (2009). Human synthetic sebum formulation and stability under conditions of use and storage. *International Journal of Cosmetic Science.* Retrieved from http://www.ncbi.nlm.nih.gov/pubmed/19134124

Zawahry, M. (MD), Hegazy, M. Rashad (MD), & Helal, M. (Bph, PhCh). (1973, January/February). Use of Aloe in treating leg ulcers and dermatoses. *International Journal of Dermatology, 12,* 68-73.

LABOR OF LOVE

Chiel, D., & Massey, L. (2001). *Curly Girl - The Handbook – A Celebration of Curls: How to cut them, care for them, love them, and set them free.* New York: Workman Publishing Company.

McKay, T. (2006). What's the Scoop on Silicones? *NaturallyCurly.com.* Retrieved from http://www.naturallycurly.com/curlreading/curly-q-a/whats-the-scoop-on-silicones

SEASONAL HAIR TIPS

McKay, T. (2009). Humidity, Humectants, and the Dew Point. *NaturallyCurly.com*. Retrieved from http://www.naturallycurly.com/curlreading/curl-products/humidity-humectants-and-the-dew-point

McKay, T. (2007), Humidity, Humectants, and Hair. *NaturallyCurly.com*. Retrieved from http://www.naturallycurly.com/curlreading/curl-products/curlchemist-humidity-humectants-and-hair

AYURVEDA

An Alternative Medicine and Complementary Medicine Resource Guide. *Alternative Medicine Foundation*. Retrieved from http://www.amfoundation.org/ayurveda.htm

Janseen, M. B. (1999). *Naturally Healthy Hair*. North Adams, MA: Storey Publishing.

Nimmannit, U., Pongrakhananon, V., & Chanvorachote, P. (2011). Emblica (*Phyllanthus emblica* Linn.) Fruit Extract Promotes Proliferation in Dermal Papilla Cells of Human Hair Follicle. Research Journal of Medicinal Plants. Retrieved from http://scialert.net/ qredirect.php?doi=rjmp.2011.95.100&linkid=pdf

Sunnydale, H. (2007). *The Complete Beauty Book*. Leicester, UK: Anness Publishing.

COLORING HAIR

Cartwright-Jones, C. (2006). Henna for Hair: "How-To" Henna. Stow, Ohio: Tap Dancing Lizard, LLC

HAIR BREAKAGE & HAIR LOSS

Fischer, T. W., Hipler, U. C., & Elsner, P. (2007). Effect of caffeine and testosterone on the proliferation of human hair follicles in vitro. International

Journal of Dermatology. Retrieved from http://www.ncbi.nlm.nih.gov/pubmed/17214716

Gathers, R., Johnson, D., Joseph, C. L. M., Kapke, A., & Wright, D. (2010). Hair Care Practices and Their Association with Scalp and Hair Disorders in African American Girls. *Journal of the American Academy of Dermatology.* Retrieved from http://www.eblue.org/article/ S0190-9622%2810%2900630-4/abstract

Gathers, R. C., & Lim, H. (2009). Central Centrifugal Cicatricial Alopecia: Past, Present, and Future. *Journal of the American Academy of Dermatology.* Retrieved from http://www.eblue.org/article/S0190-9622%2808%2901444-8/abstract

Hantash, B., M.D., Ph.D. (2011). Scarring Alopecia. *Medscape Reference.* Retrieved from http://emedicine.medscape.com/article/1073559-overview

Hay, I., Jamieson, M., & Ormerod, A. (1998). Randomized Trial of Aromatherapy – Successful Treatment for Alopecia. Archives of Dermatology. Retrieved from http://archderm.ama-assn.org/ cgi/content/short/134/11/1349

CPSIA information can be obtained
at www.ICGtesting.com
Printed in the USA
LVOW04s2138280616

494502LV00010B/148/P